Revisiting HIV/AIDS in French Culture

Revisiting HIV/AIDS in French Culture

Raw Matters

Edited by Loïc Bourdeau
and V. Hunter Capps

LEXINGTON BOOKS
Lanham • Boulder • New York • London

Published by Lexington Books
An imprint of The Rowman & Littlefield Publishing Group, Inc.
4501 Forbes Boulevard, Suite 200, Lanham, Maryland 20706
www.rowman.com

86-90 Paul Street, London EC2A 4NE

British Library Cataloguing in Publication Information Available

Library of Congress Cataloging-in-Publication Data Available

ISBN 978-1-7936-5008-5 (cloth)
ISBN 978-1-7936-5009-2 (electronic)

To those we have lost to AIDS and those left behind
who still carry the weight of these losses.

Contents

Acknowledgments

This project would not have been possible without the enthusiastic response we received from our invited contributors. We would like to thank them. They are (in order of appearance): David Caron, Daniel. N. Maroun, Brian Troth, João Florêncio, Lucille Toth, and CJ Gomolka. We also want to thank Nicholas Giguère and Kevin Lambert who agreed to take part in our interview. It has been a pleasure to collaborate with everyone, to learn from their scholarship. Along the way we have created a new space of discussion, debate, and support.

Loïc Bourdeau: Thinking back to the early years of the epidemic—I was born in France the year that "AIDS" was officially coined—I realized I did not know anything about the crisis. I had never heard of it until I was 7 when French actress Clémentine Célarié appeared on the first televised fundraiser (Sidaction) and kissed HIV+ Patrice Janiaud to debunk myths around transmission. This moment struck me and is still part of French television history. Except for the annual fundraiser, I still didn't hear much about it. In middle school, however, my two best friends (Aurélie and Clarisse) and I chose to do our biology research project on HIV/AIDS (Clarisse's father was a doctor of infectious disease at our city hospital). I am thankful for this first foray into medicine, which has guided my career. While I work in the humanities, care and healthcare remain central concerns as they are deeply linked to equity, diversity, social justice, and politics. I would also like to thank my department at the University of Louisiana at Lafayette, which generously supports my research and allows me to be part of an international network of amazing scholars. Meeting Hunter in London, UK, in 2018 has renewed my passion for research and collaboration. I thank him for working on this volume and other projects with me.

V. Hunter Capps: I would like to thank the academic community at the University at Buffalo, specifically Amy Graves Monroe and the Department of Comparative Literature. As always, I must give thanks to my grandfather Joseph Kern for being an unwavering supporter of all that I do. I would also like to thank those who have helped keep me going: Anjanette, Kathleen, Anthony, and Brian. Without you girls, I simply would not be here. To the French singer Leslie who was the catalyst for my endeavors into the francophone world. For my baby, Roger, who left me too soon. Thank you for giving me the love you could while you were here. And a big thanks to Loïc for putting theory into practice by fostering queer community and care in academic spaces.

Finally, we would like to extend a very special thank you to David Caron whose scholarship has been and is so influential and inspiring to us and to the field of (French) HIV/AIDS studies. Reading his work is always a very singular and enriching experience, and we are so honored that he agreed to contribute a chapter to this volume.

Introduction

Revisiting Sites of Rawness, Queerness, and Vulnerability

Loïc Bourdeau and V. Hunter Capps

Revisiting HIV/AIDS in French Culture: Raw Matters is about encounters and relations. It is the result of a network of collaboration between scholars who share interests in HIV/AIDS cultural studies, as well as in questions of equality, diversity, and social justice. First and foremost, this volume owes much to the *120 BPM Symposium* held in London, UK (May 2019) where we (Bourdeau and Capps) first met and gave talks on Robin Campillo's 2017 hit film. Set in 1990s France, *120 BPM* (or *BPM*) follows "the grassroots political organization Act Up-Paris (AIDS Coalition to Unleash Power) and its members as they react to government apathy in the face of rising death tolls and the medical establishment's slow efforts at finding a cure" (Capps 2018). Following the conference, we continued to exchange about the current resurgence of French cultural productions dealing with the 1980s and 1990s HIV/AIDS crisis, wondering why the contemporary moment was propitious to new cultural explorations. Indeed, while Campillo's film has received much critical acclaim and drawn attention at an international level, it is but one example of a larger phenomenon in the post–2010 French landscape. Other productions include, among others, Jean-Philippe Amar's *Pilules Bleues* [*Blue Pills*] (2015), Vincent Boujon's *Vivant!* [*Alive!*] (2015), Olivier Ducastel and Jacques Martineau's *Théo et Hugo dans le même bateau* [*Paris 5:59: Theo and Hugo*] (2016), Christophe Honoré's *Plaire, aimer et courir vite* [*Sorry Angels*] (2018) along with his play *Les Idoles* [*Idols*] (2019), and even, to some extent, Alain Guiraudie's earlier *L'inconnu du lac* [*Stranger by the Lake*] (2013).[1] Forty years after the first official case of AIDS, the current proliferation of productions that tackle the painful history thus seems to attest to a need to testify, to speak up, and to put a end to France's cultural amnesia, especially as the world experiences another pandemic. As

CJ Gomolka notes in his contribution to this volume, and as we also do in another contribution about the languages of COVID (an international project led by Piotr Blumczynski and Steven Wilson), France's response to the spread of SARV-CoV-2 has reopened an old wound—or rather, has rubbed salt in a wound that has yet to heal. Declaring to the nation that "Cette épidémie . . . est la plus grave crise sanitaire qu'ait connu la France depuis un siècle ["This epidemic . . . is the most serious health crisis that France has experienced in over a century"] (2020)," President Emmanuel Macron discounted the 30,000+ individual lives that died of AIDS-related complications a few decades ago, as well as the lives that are still lost today to the disease. Though numbers are decreasing over time, in 2020 alone, "1.5 million individuals worldwide acquired HIV" and "690,000 people died from AIDS-related illnesses" (HIV.gov 2021). Or as Jih-Fei Cheng, Alexandra Juhasz, and Nishant Shahani write: "AIDS remains the longest enduring modern pandemic without a cure and without widespread access to preventative care or treatment for the majority of those infected with HIV" (2020, 3). This volume thus emerges in a context of cultural revitalization *and* during a pandemic caused by "a new microbial killer" (Greenfeld 2020); a new pandemic that has once again challenged governmental, media, healthcare, and linguistic responses.

Yet, as much as COVID-19 has taken over our personal and academic lives—several chapters connect both pandemics as we do here—it bears keeping in mind that this project predates the outbreak and is first inscribed in a broader movement to excavate the past, to shed light once more, to revisit (i.e., to look at things from a different angle) the 1980s and 1990s crisis along with its more recent cultural iterations. Beyond the foundational texts that inform this introduction and each chapter—and to which we owe our larger debt—recent scholarship attests to lasting interests and ongoing developments in the field. In "Introduction: The Show Must Go On: HIV/AIDS and Queer Studies in Twenty-First-Century France," Maxime Foerster and Daniel Maroun ask what it means to study HIV/AIDS today, whether we are "doomed to solely focus on the past" (2021, 121), and note that "now we understand better that 'the AIDS crisis is not over,' because we renew each voice and each testimony as we witness them, study them, and give them the stage bringing the periphery to the center" (125). Our endeavor lies in a similar attempt to connect past and present, to continue to unearth voices, lived experiences, and lessons that can help us shape a better future. Cheng et al.'s aforementioned volume, *AIDS and the Distribution of Crises*, further reminds us that "it matters where we locate the crises, how we temporalize their multiple durations, and when and how we identify, name, categorize their impacts" (2020, 4). In our case, we have elected to focus solely on the French context from the onset of the epidemic to today. At times, we turn to France's transatlantic neighbor, the United States, not only because they have a long political history and were the most impacted (in the West) by HIV, but also because the entire political response to AIDS in France was based on an American template, which, in turn, troubled the French model. Other recent publications, such as Chase Ledin's "Retroactivism and Futurity in *120 BPM* and *Théo et Hugo*" (2021) or João Florêncio's *Bareback Porn, Porous Masculinities, Queer Futures; The Ethics of Becoming-Pig* (2020) also examine, respectively, how AIDS activism is presented in today's cultural productions, and how gay masculinities and gay erotic culture have changed with the advent of antiretroviral therapies.

We are part of a larger and lively discussion. In our case "raw" or "rawness" has become a new site of investigation, a new way to contribute to this discussion. In an interview about *BPM*, Campillo—who was an active member of Act Up-Paris—remembers: "We all ran through those years disconnected from our emotions . . . I was very used to going to hospital. When I opened the door to a hospital room I knew how to behave for the person on the bed. For them not to see my emotions was conditional. I went in with a stern face, speaking very simply. It meant we were all very disconnected" (Shepherd 2018). In directing *BPM*, Campillo sought to expose the trauma and the historical wounds, while reconnecting with the raw emotions he did not have a chance to process. He also reconnected our present to the past, urging us, if not to remember, to learn from these raw and vulnerable times. Four decades earlier, seropositive queer writers took up the shifting landscape of identity, community, and sexual desire in the wake of AIDS and its ravages in order to both make new subjectivities brought about by HIV/AIDS intelligible, as well as to harness the inherently democratic space of literature for the exploration and critique of the status quo. They utilized the particular genre of autofiction to put on raw display the suffering, trauma, anxieties, pleasure, and bonding that took place in light of the crisis. The raw quality of their writing, from the content to the form, exemplified the shock waves from AIDS that still today affect the manner in which we approach and understand queerness. As such, cultural productions have always aided in defining the parameters of the epidemic. In this volume we ask what this idea of rawness, born from strictly queer sexual practices and later deployed through art forms, can do for evolving conversations about queerness in France. What are the implications of rawness with respect to the project of writing and literature, but also cinema and the arts, as it serves a broader political project? Understanding "raw" as etymologically linked to the Latin "crudus" and thus also encompassing the crude, how does queerness and its transgressive tendencies manifest through cultural productions? In shifting the sociopolitical landscape of French democracy, how do ruminations on HIV/AIDS challenge heteronormative standards of citizenship, and what has been/should be the role that the arts play therein? As we revisit, we raise new questions, highlight new modes of sociality, and new queer-world making possibilities.

EARLY AIDS DISCOURSE

How does one begin to assess AIDS cultural productions without attacking head on exactly what AIDS means? Many writers from a variety of disciplines have taken up the task of attempting to describe and explain the complex social and biomedical disaster that was the AIDS crisis, all with varying degrees of input that have produced a rich body of literature that ranges from social theory to the biomedical. Taking into account much of this literature, our interests focus specifically on the Western interpretation of the epidemic as it pertains to its early unfolding as a gay disease, how the disease gave shape to a nascent gay community, and how that community was affected by and responded to the AIDS crisis. Furthermore, HIV/AIDS played a role in the then-developing ideas of queerness and how its resonance is still felt today. In order to explore this relationship between AIDS and queerness, it is necessary to look at the writings of those most disproportionately affected by the epidemic. While AIDS as a pandemic can be approached from several angles, it would be beyond the scope of this volume to attempt to assess the disease outside the reach of the Western phenomenon more specifically implicated in the utterance of the "AIDS crisis," and though its global and relative perspectives are far from mutually exclusive we seek to examine the ways in which the disease as a social crisis has shifted queer thought pertaining to sex, desire, and subjectivity.

1981 is regarded as the first year of the epidemic in both North America and France. This year is designated as such due to the medical community taking notice of a small cluster of opportunistic infections as well as depleted immune systems in otherwise healthy gay men in urban locations such as New York City, San Francisco, and Paris. In the years that followed, the medical community and the then-infantile gay community scrambled to find answers as the death toll began to quickly rise with little to no response or recognition by the government. In those early days, due to both a lack of knowledge concerning the disease as well as a seemingly benign association with those most affected by the disease, what we now know as AIDS was first labeled GRID (gay-related immune deficiency). By 1982, an epidemiological cluster study conducted in Los Angeles attempted to demonstrate that the disease, by then already labeled AIDS (acquired immune deficiency syndrome), was sexually transmissible. Though the study has long since been critiqued for its narrow scope, two-dimensional framework, and its dry, scientific assessment of human relations, the study speaks to the early manner in which the disease was explicitly linked with gay men and their sexual practices. Indeed, this study was the basis upon which Randy Shilts built his sensationalized account of "Patient Zero," the infamously beautiful Gaétan Dugas who was labeled as "O" for Outside-of-California in the study. This "O" went through several phases of interpretation that coupled with the desperate drive of a journalist produced the popular, best-selling novel *And the Band Played On* (1987) wherein Shilts ran wild with the reading of the "O" as "0," and as they say, the rest is history.

In taking up the project of conducting research with respect to AIDS, one must confront the overwhelmingly layered nature of the phenomenon that this outdated moniker represents. In one respect, the acronym AIDS was born in 1982 after it replaced its passively homophobic antecedent GRID and denotes a syndrome marked by a decrease in white blood cells as well as the presence of one or many opportunistic infections. Although in 1987, after a scientific, cultural, and political clash between American and French doctors, AIDS was replaced by HIV, the new name for the retrovirus that caused the syndrome, "AIDS" still pervaded language and thought in a manner that the acronym has to this day permeated any framing of the illness. Presently, AIDS most literally is used to mark a threshold of 200 CD4 cells per cubic millimeter of blood. However, AIDS as a concept has come to represent much more than this simple biological marker. The word *AIDS* was and still is highly associated with gay men which speaks to the political history of the word, for AIDS was never simply a biomedical crisis that had to do with a virus; it was from the very start a political and cultural crisis that saw those most disproportionately affected bear the stigma of the disease alongside bearing the weight of friends and lovers lost en masse.

Early AIDS discourse sought to grapple with how conceptions of the disease emerged as well as what those conceptions meant for the ongoing epidemic at large. In real time, scientists, cultural critics, and activists were investing themselves in the processes of meaning making surrounding the disease and those affected by it. Paula Treichler's *How to Have Theory in an Epidemic: Cultural Chronicles of AIDS*, a collection of essays from the 1980s and 1990s, did the necessary work of demonstrating how important it was for scholars at the time to critically examine the mechanisms and methods that produced cultural understandings of the disease with particular emphasis in some parts on biomedical discourse and its claim to objectivity. Her work on AIDS discourse is the pivotal starting point from which this study grounds its understanding of "AIDS" at all. In the prologue to the collection of essays, Treichler frames the larger text by summarily saying that "the AIDS epidemic has produced a parallel epidemic of meanings, definitions, and attributions . . . *an epidemic of signification* . . . The AIDS epidemic is cultural and linguistic as well as biological and biomedical"

(1999, 1, emphasis in original). Later, she notes: "The very nature of AIDS is constructed through language and in particular through discourses of medicine and science . . . The name *AIDS* in part *constructs* the disease and helps make it intelligible" (11, emphasis in original). In short, from a baseline starting point, this study takes AIDS to represent a signifier of multiple sociocultural and biomedical phenomena that at times coalesce discursively enough to be better understood but that also at times come into conflict with their inner workings. It is because of this double-edged sword of discursive amorphousness and malleability that we wish to pay special linguistic attention to the deployment of different terms in this study such as HIV, AIDS, sida, etc. As researchers observing and engaging with AIDS-related discourse and language, we cannot and do not seek to concretize exactly what AIDS is per se. Instead, we seek to examine most broadly what AIDS as a biomedical and sociopolitical crisis has meant for institutions of democracy, literature, culture, and queerness.

With disciplinary leanings in art history and art criticism, scholar and activist Douglas Crimp was also an early contributor to the field of AIDS discourse. In 1987, Crimp edited and contributed to an AIDS-specific edition of the journal *October* titled *AIDS: Cultural Analysis/Cultural Activism*. In his eponymous essay, Crimp's main argument was that art and activism were cultural practices germane to the project of understanding AIDS. He explains: "AIDS does not exist apart from the practices that conceptualize it, represent it, and respond to it. We know AIDS only in and through those practices" (2). He concludes as well that "AIDS intersects with and requires a critical rethinking of all of culture: of language and representation, of science and medicine, of health and illness, of sex and death, of the public and private realms" (15). Crimp speaks in rather totalizing terms in his early assessment of exactly what AIDS represented, and his assertions concerning how AIDS required a revamping or reworking of social structures and thought were indeed an accurate judgment that acknowledged how powerful AIDS was. Furthermore, Crimp's essay emphasized that it was for these very reasons that activists, artists, and those most affected by the disease undertook the sociocultural work of helping shape how AIDS was constructed and perceived since it was a virulently homophobic and heteronormative public that was exploiting and sensationalizing the epidemic all to the detriment of the HIV-positive.

In *Policing Desire: Pornography, AIDS, and the Media*, Simon Watney remarks, "Aids [sic] is not only a medical crisis on an unparalleled scaled, it involves a crisis of representation itself, a crisis over the entire framing of knowledge about the human body and its capacities for sexual pleasure" (1987, 9). Nearly verbatim, Watney echoes Treichler in asserting just how critical AIDS was with respect to the social mechanisms that produce meaning.

However, these three early AIDS discourse writers also paid special attention to the component of the epidemic that had to do with those most affected by it. On this point, Watney says, "Thus, whilst individuals are vulnerable to HIV infection, the entire reproductive machinery of gay subjectivity is also vulnerable to the ideological fall-out of the representational crisis triggered by the virus" (18). He cites gay subjectivity here to acknowledge how gay men were not only bearing the brunt of the disease. At the same time, AIDS itself was affecting discourse on queerness, although Watney, in a clear nod to Foucault, calls it the "pejorative discourse of 'homosexuality' with the familiar connotations of effeminacy, contagion and degeneracy" (18).

Watney is not the only scholar who acknowledged this connection with AIDS and the evolving discourse on queerness, but his articulation of that connection contextualizes the sense of AIDS that we seek to develop with respect to this volume as a whole. To summarize, early AIDS discourse labored to demonstrate how it was that a disease caused by a virus that affected certain minority groups of people, who were blamed and neglected because of political and moral leanings, in fact ruptured and required a revamping of social mechanisms of knowledge production and meaning making. If gay liberation had preceded AIDS, it was AIDS that would define queerness' parameters from here on out. For the purposes of this volume, what needs to be gleaned from this early discourse is that AIDS marked a significant cultural shift for queers that necessitated new definitions of queerness as much as it necessitated, and perhaps even birthed, the critical thinking that underscores queer thought itself. In other words, "AIDS" underlies any sense of "queerness" at all.

RAWNESS, RISK, AND VULNERABILITY

Rather early on in the epidemic, scientists were able to determine that HIV was sexually transmissible. Sex then took center stage when it came to any coverage or discussion of the disease. America saw the rise of Larry Kramer, most notably known for creating the Gay Men's Health Crisis (GMHC), the first community-based AIDS service provider, as well as having a hand in the early organizing of ACT UP, the AIDS Coalition to Unleash Power. However, central to Kramer's early approaches was a particularly anti-sex discourse that actually predated HIV's emergence onto the gay scene of the 1980s as seen in his first novel *Faggots* (1978) which offered a scathing criticism of the promiscuous, drug-fueled gay scene of the 1970s. With the rise of pre-exposure prophylaxis (PrEP) in 2012 that showed a significant efficacy in reducing HIV transmission rates, Kramer stubbornly continued to rely on this anti-sex discourse as he remarked that taking the drug to prevent HIV was "cowardly" (Healy 2014). A few years later, in 2016, he added:

> I'm not grateful for having lost hundreds of friends, and I never forget them. I'm not grateful that gay people still are leading—many of us—lives that got us into the same kind of mess that we got into in '81. They're relaxing their sense of responsibility and having unsafe sex. And because of this PrEP stuff, which is certainly helpful, people are using it as an excuse to go back and have the crazy sex lives we had in the disco days, and we mustn't do that. ("36 years and counting" 2017)

By framing his sentiments as not being grateful, Kramer foregrounds his dissatisfaction with the immense number of friends that he lost to the epidemic. However, in the same breath, he effectively blames those very friends whose losses he mourns by citing their sexual practices as the reason for the spread of HIV. Indeed, he draws a direct line of culpability from those who died in the '80s and '90s to those taking PrEP today. The only acknowledgment of PrEP's efficacy comes in the form of a brief and passing "certainly helpful" but not before Kramer quickly adds that promiscuity is still the culprit responsible for HIV. To summarize, Christophe Broqua most succinctly observed about Kramer that, "He would subsequently condemn those [gay] lifestyles tirelessly and vocally, especially when they no longer appeared to comply as strictly with preventative standards" ([2005] 2020, 229).

Kramer's actions provide a glimpse of how the stigma surrounding gay sex existed within the gay community itself and was central to the conversations about AIDS at the time. Given the specifically French nature of this volume, it may seem odd to begin with an American activist. However, it was Kramer and the American model of activism and organizing that French activists later used as a template for Act Up-Paris. The original ACT UP had its first protest in March of 1987 as the group performed a die-in at the intersection of Broadway and Wall Street in order to disrupt traffic and bring attention to the apathy and inaction toward AIDS. It was not until 1989 that Act Up-Paris was born. Broqua notes in his history on the group: "Beyond mobilization on AIDS, Act-Up-Paris claimed the legacy of what members called 'gay activism' whose birth is precisely dated and celebrated each year in Gay Pride events across the world" (33). As such, he historically and politically links Act Up-Paris with a particularly American-inflected queer model of politics and activism. Didier Lestrade, one of Act Up-Paris's co-founders, was especially forthright in his admiration of Larry Kramer, and thus it would come as no surprise that Lestrade became just as infamous for his vitriolic discourse on gay sex in particular.[2]

After the arrival of successful antiretroviral therapy for HIV in 1996, France saw the emergence of the barebacking debates. On the one side were the authors Guillaume Dustan and Erik Rémès who had written books and made public appearances in the media to defend the practices of condomless sex, otherwise known as raw sex, among HIV-positive gay men. On the other side was Didier Lestrade and other members of Act Up-Paris who argued that these authors represented a dangerous "relapse" back into behavior that was irresponsible and to blame for the spread of HIV. At stake in this debate was not simply the definition of individual sexual liberty and autonomy but rather the raison d'être of Act Up-Paris at all. As Oliver Davis notes, "The operation against the bareback writers was the first time Act-Up had turned its formidable war-machine against individuals acting in a personal capacity and, moreover, against people who, as HIV-positive gay men, shared the same combination of three defining identity traits with those whom Lestrade envisaged as the groups' own constituency" (2015, 147). In short, Lestrade and Act Up-Paris's sights shifted away from the government and were set upon those most impacted by the epidemic. However, more than just an assault on HIV-positive individuals and their risk-informed practices, "Act Up's refusal to recognize Dustan's claim to the freedom of literary space was its first coercive strike against not just this particular writer, but against the institution of literature and the ideal of democracy it embodies" (146).

It is here where we might arrive at the heart of what this volume seeks to explore. From the beginning of the epidemic, sex was on trial. More to the point, gay sex was being reified as the culprit responsible for disease and degeneracy it had always been portrayed to be not only by the media and the political right, but also by similar discourse espoused by those like Kramer and Lestrade. For the bareback writers, the debate began with the HIV-positive since among each other condoms no longer served a purpose in preventing HIV infection. Soon thereafter however, Dustan and Rémès made it clear that their philosophy on barebacking extended to the sexual practices of *all* people regardless of their serostatus. The simple logic was that one's choice to abandon prophylactics should not be a basis upon which to ground a moralization of sexual practices. They sought to demonstrate how risk itself was part and parcel of sexual desire and that everyone must negotiate that risk by their own metrics. Furthermore, to frame HIV infection as indicative of an individual's moral failure is ultimately the basis upon which people could blame gay men for their infections and the epidemic writ large. This rhetoric of blame relied upon and fortified a discourse of homosexuality as an inherently depraved illness, which in turn is what propped up governmental indifference and discrimination. In truth, what the bareback writers were ultimately arguing for was an embrasure of the very thing that had once been a site of joy and community making, but that was stripped from them because of disease and death. They sought not a naïve return to a pre-AIDS world but rather to build a new one where one could be HIV-positive *and* gay men could still enjoy the unfettered pleasures of sex.

If it is one thing to consider a sense of liberty to choose one's sexual practices, we must do so by revisiting some of the fundamentals of democracy. To center sex in this conversation is to bring to the fore some of the most essential democratic elements that AIDS as a phenomenon radically altered. The topic and practice of sex is often relegated to the realm of the private given its intimate nature. However, this relegation to the private has not stopped governments from intervening in attempts to control how and where sex takes place as much as define what sex is for. Because HIV disproportionately affected homosexual men, the disease was quickly associated with the so-labeled deviant sexual behavior practiced by these men. As the heterosexual population became infected, then and only then did the state deem the problem one of the "general public." ACT UP brought attention to how France and America denied public attention, care, and resources to their citizens and justified doing so with an appeal to the private/public separation in democratic society. The plural sexual and identitarian politics that were so intimate with the emergence of the AIDS crisis contested the boundaries of how and where the state should act in a democratic manner that bestows all of its citizens with equal dignity and respect. In France where the model of republicanism relies on racial, religious, and sexual difference being relegated to the private sphere so that the French citizen might remain constant, secular, and "equal," gay men and others saw themselves neglected by the country that vowed to protect them. David Caron echoes this point when he states that, "As the epidemiology of AIDS tells us, a community *was* there, but its political inexistence made any effective response impossible" (2014, 160, emphasis in original). Thus, when a sexually transmitted disease began infecting a sexual minority population, the fight for rights and dignity required moving away from a moralizing discourse of individual responsibility and moving toward a discourse that critically examined the role of sex in the constitution of democratic rights and citizenship. Simply put, sex became a public good.

In Judith Butler's 2004 essay *Violence, Mourning, Politics*, she provides an analysis that helps to elucidate the complex affective and political web in which activists and loved ones were caught during the AIDS crisis. She writes:

> We tend to narrate the history of the feminist and lesbian/gay movement, for instance, in such a way that ecstasy figured prominently in the sixties and seventies and midway through the eighties . . . To be ecstatic means, literally, to be outside oneself, and thus can have several meanings: to be transported beyond oneself by a passion, but also to be *beside oneself* with rage or grief. I think that

> if I can still address a "we,'" or include myself within its terms, I am speaking to those of us who are living in certain ways *beside ourselves*, whether in sexual passion, or emotional grief, or political rage. (24, emphasis in original)

Grasping the political dimensions of sex in a world after the emergence of HIV is a rather simple task, but as Butler notes, the political sits on a spectrum with other affective dimensions. As lovers and friends continued to die, those left behind had to grapple with incomprehensible loss and immense grief. Once a pleasurable gesture of sharing ecstasy and community building, sex also became a harbinger of death. Enraged by political neglect, crippled by the emotional toll of what Dagmawi Woubshet has called rapid and "compounding loss" (2015, 1), and still nevertheless staking a claim to a new kind of sexual citizenship is the complex intersection where queer people found themselves in the tumult of the AIDS crisis. Indeed, these intense emotions became less discernible from each other as activists harnessed their grief into political protest. Such was the case with political funerals that consisted of activists marching their deceased loved ones through the streets. Activists also participated in the Ashes Action during which they marched to the White House and spread the ashes of their deceased loved ones on the lawn. Death and mourning, typically private matters in the West, became public, and in doing so activists were able to make it difficult for anyone to avert their eyes from the crude injustices of AIDS. Douglas Crimp remarks in his essay "Mourning and Militancy" that "Alongside the dismal toll of death, what many of us have lost is a culture of sexual possibility: back rooms, tea rooms, bookstores, movie houses, and baths; the trucks, the pier, the ramble, the dunes" (1989, 140). It was not simply the deaths, as if those losses were not enough, that those left behind had to mourn, but they also had to mourn the loss of a queer world that was once overbrimming with sexual potentiality. It is worth noting here that in discussing AIDS, we must also resist a nostalgia for a pre-AIDS time as if AIDS alone were responsible for diminishing an otherwise perfect world. To do so would be to play into a fable that is constructed by and through Western notions of whiteness. AIDS and the trauma it wrought, then, should be understood not as some revolutionary calamity that produced conditions that were unlivable but rather as yet another chapter in a longer history of Western exploitation, colonialism, slavery, and genocide.

Ann Cvetkovich tells us that "Trauma then serves as a site for exploring the convergence of affect and sexuality as categories of analysis for queer theory" (2003, 48). From political funerals to the military metaphor, AIDS wrought a new kind of trauma into queer history. Nevertheless, queers continued to harness this trauma in generative ways as sex became a collective political gesture that queers taking up as a praxis so as to establish a new kind of sociality, a new community, a new future. Over time, these interwoven affects have been intergenerationally transmitted[3] through the mediums of art, literature, and sex itself.[4] Juana María Rodríguez argues that gestures "are inflected by the scent and sense of cultures marked by time, yet they also traverse borders and resist temporal categorization" (2014, 4) and furthers this point by noting that "Queer gestures are those that highlight the everyday labor of political, social, and sexual energies that mark our collective will to survive this day, or to at least make the effort" (8). In this context, "queer" emphasizes the role of process, collectivity, survival, and the everyday laboring required for existing at all. As such, we can see how contemporary queers are taking up the mantel with PrEP by embracing vulnerability and risk in the name of a political project that exceeds them alone. PrEP functions as a reaching out across space and time, a continued queering of temporality in step with the political and social projects of the queer ancestors lost to the epidemic that works to not only ease the ontological weight of this trauma but that also fortifies queer models of kinship.[5] PrEP users actually reach out and take responsibility, help shoulder the burden of the epidemic that has heretofore weighed so heavily on our HIV-positive queer forbearers.[6] This gesture leans toward a sense of community that began with the Stonewall riots and was further buttressed during the AIDS crisis. We can thus understand how AIDS has shaped and continues to shape the contours of queerness, that amorphous term whose discursive purpose was born from centering sexuality as a new basis of analyzing the parameters of the human.

David Caron aptly observes that "If the self doesn't preexist the contract but is instead an effect of it, then selfhood is contracted, like a virus or other foreign body, thanks to the unplanned encounters or because, for whatever reason, we let our guard down" (2014, 86). It is in this context then that we ought to imagine what might happen or what might it look like if we permanently let our guard down? What if we lay bare our raw emotions and have raw sex at the risk of losing ourselves in the process? While it may be possible to mitigate our exposure to both viruses and others, it is utterly impossible to protect ourselves entirely should we seek to live a life at all. During the AIDS crisis, a virus was purposefully left to ravage undesirable communities who turned around and utilized that political exploitation and vulnerability to foster care and love for each other. Now, during COVID-19, calls for collective unity in augmenting our lives are front and center. We are seemingly embracing this shared vulnerability to each other so as to work together in ending this pandemic by, ironically enough, isolating ourselves from each other. However, will this heightened attention to our shared vulnerability dissipate? In other words, when will the mythic "general public" be able to return to public gatherings and places without the fear of a silent and deadly virus lying just beyond our perception? How will the "general public" ever be able to not pay manic attention to our exposure to each other? It is our hope that despite the repeated failings of government to maintain and protect its citizenry "we" are able to learn from this experience and not regress to a time and place where we fortify that which separates us.

CHAPTER BREAKDOWN

This volume comprises eight chapters and opens with David Caron's "Transmitting It: Rawness and the Politics of HIV/AIDS Witnessing Today." One of the leading figures in (French) AIDS studies, Caron argues that AIDS writing (past and present) carries the potential for disruption and for breaking the silence that has and continues to undermine the traumatic nature of the epidemic. Looking to both sides of the Atlantic (France and the United States) and engaging with older and more recent cultural productions, this chapter engages with questions of memory, denial, and testimony to show that HIV/AIDS is still relevant today, that raw writing comes with great political force, and that testifying is first and foremost about injustice. The wounds will remain raw and will continue to haunt us, for the better. In the following chapter, "Raw Writing: AIDS Autofiction and the Construction of Seropositive Subjectivity," V. Hunter Capps explores raw writing, that is, a genre or style of writing deployed by queer and seropositive individuals (such as Hervé Guibert and Guillaume Dustan) who utilized queer excess in the form of sex, the body, language, and drugs to make intelligible new subjectivities brought about by HIV. Overall, Capps's goal is to demonstrate how such writing and those behind it helped to elaborate on and spread new forms of queer knowledge that have reshaped the parameters of sex, desire, and communities. In "Kindling Kinships: Sexual Citizenship and Queer Constructions of Masculinity in the Works of Erik Rémès," Daniel N. Maroun engages with another key figures of AIDS writing and argues that Rémès empowers the queer notions of sexual citizenship that are grounded in the effacement of heterosexuality from his novel as his protagonists seroconvert both tertiary characters and the readers themselves. This process of seroconversion repopulates his literary worlds and establishes a queer lineage, a bloodline that mimics heterosexual concepts of *filiation*. For Maroun, Rémès uses the serostatus of his protagonists to reach a goal: breeding a queer literary universe via disease transmission and re-anchoring queer seropositive masculinity in a much more classical and raw concept of seed spreading. This interpretation highlights how this queer performance of masculinity aligns with heterosexual concepts of French republican duty. Brian Troth's "Covering Up: Condomless Sex, (Ir)responsibility, and Risk in France" turns to Rémès, Dustan, and more recent productions and argues that barebacking and condomless sex perturb cultural norms of responsible sexual behavior and responsible behavior in the midst of a pandemic. While opponents have frequently vilified barebacking and condomless sex as irresponsible, advances in medication such as effective Antiretroviral Treatment (ART) and pre-exposure prophylaxis (PrEP) allow for certain "dangerous" sexual behaviors to occur without infection. We should then reassess risk and redefine responsibility. Troth tempers his analysis with the inclusion of public sexual health campaigns from the 1990s and the mid- to late-2010s. This chapter fulfills a need to reconsider and reassess the processes by which we choose to protect ourselves and what, if anything, constitutes "risky" behavior. In "'C'est Votre Choix' or, Private Identities and Public Militancy in the Second Decade of the AIDS Epidemic in France: The Case of Gay Porn Magazine *Projet X*," João Florêncio shows how historians of the gay movement have tended to privilege activist records and publications thus overlooking erotic and pornographic media as sources in their telling of how a community came together as a politicized critical mass (Florêncio and Miller 2022). The same phenomenon is also to be encountered in existing cultural histories of HIV and AIDS. Florêncio looks at the history of the French gay hardcore magazine *Projet X* (1994–2000) to shine some much-needed light on the complex and often contradictory manner in which gay men—and subcultural gay sex media—responded to the AIDS crisis. In the end, this chapters adds to the growing literature that complicates the myth of immediate and generalized condom adherence among gay men in the aftermath of AIDS. The last two chapters in this volume deal more directly with HIV/AIDS and the ongoing SARS-CoV-2/COVID-19 pandemic. Lucille Toth, in "Viral Dances: Moving in Times of a Pandemic," investigates three main epidemics, from the Saint Vitus' dancing plagues in 16th-century France to the HIV/AIDS crisis and viral TikTok Tok in the COVID-19 era. In this chapter, Toth discusses the informative, educative, and political roles of dance as these epidemics generate(d) cultural productions that question the cross-history of dance and contamination. Confronting dance with the idea of virality will allow us to confront the medical humanities with political dance theories in order to reevaluate the legacy of AIDS in the field of French studies. The last academic chapter, by CJ Gomolka, "State of Sexual Exception: SARS-CoV-2, HIV, and Sexual Citizenship in Pandemic Times," connects both crises and shows how the specter of the AIDS crisis was redeployed within the mediatized discursive grid that attempted to bring some type of intelligibility to the SARS-CoV-2 pandemic and its global effects. In particular, Gomolka analyzes the effects of these epidemiological comparisons, the crude conspiracy theories, and the ways sociopolitical actors mobilized queer sociosexual practices and pulled from S/M sartorial play in conversations about risk reduction during sex. As such, the chapter offers new understandings of the epistemologies and biotechnologies that form and inform relations between disease, sex, subject, and citizenship. Finally, the last contribution to this volume is an interview with two millennial queer writers from Quebec, Canada: Nicholas Giguère and Kevin Lambert. Here, John Ashburn and Loïc Bourdeau ask them about their writing practice, how rawness informs their work, and their relationship with the AIDS crisis.

The act of conducting research on a pandemic that has yet to come to a close all the while another pandemic rages on feels incredibly daunting. In line with queer thought that seeks not to homogenize or solidify itself, we hesitate to offer solutions so much as we wish to frame this volume as imaginative possibilities that tap into the potential to reshape and rethink the social fabric that entwines us. This volume is itself a culmination of not only individual research and writing but also the projects of those who have come before us. As such, we offer up this volume as a collaborative one, an affective gesture predicated on archiving those whose lives live on as singular traces in art, literature, and feelings. We invite you the reader, the one who will read this study and be responsible for giving it life, animating it as well as those within it, to hold it with care, respect, and courage. In doing so, it is our hope, that we can work together to bear witness to those lost to the AIDS crisis all the while imagining and constructing more livable lives for each other.

BIBLIOGRAPHY

"37 years and counting: AIDS in America." 2017. CBC News, June 4. https://www.cbsnews.com/news/36-years-and-counting-aids-in-america/ (accessed 20 December 2021).

Broqua, Christophe. 2020 [2005]. *Action = Vie. A History of AIDS Activism and Gay Politics in France*. Philadelphia, PA: Temple University Press.

Butler, Judith. 2004. *Precarious Life: The Powers of Mourning and Violence.* New York: Verso.

Capps, V. Hunter. 2018. "A Small Movement with a Big Agenda: Robin Campillo's *BPM*." *Fiction and Film Scholars of France* 8, 5. https://h-france.net/fffh/maybe-missed/a-small-movement-with-a-big-agenda-robin-campillos-bpm/ (accessed November 2021).

Caron, David. 2014. *The Nearness of Others*. Minneapolis: University of Minnesota Press.

———. 2014. "Truvada, mon amour." *The Brooklyn Quarterly*. http://brooklynquarterly.org/truvada-mon-amour (accessed November 2021).

Cheng, Jih-Fei, Alexandra Juhasz, and Nishant Shahani (eds.). 2020. *AIDS and the Distribution of Crises*. Durham, NC: Duke University Press.

Crimp, Douglas. 1987. "AIDS: Cultural Analysis, Cultural Activism." *October*, 43: 3–16. https://doi.org/10.2307/3397562.

———. 1989. "Mourning and Militancy." *October*, 51: 3–18 https://doi.org/10.2307/778889.

Cvetkovitch, Ann. 2003. *An Archive of Feelings: Trauma, Sexuality, and Lesbian Public Cultures*. Durham, NC: Duke University Press.

Davis, Oliver. 2015. "Leading by Example: A Queer Critique of Personalization and Coercive Community Governance in ACT UP-Paris' Operation Against the Bareback Writers." *Sexualities*, 18(1/2): 141–157.

Florêncio, João. 2020. *Bareback Porn, Porous Masculinities, Queer Futures: The Ethics of Becoming-Pig*. London: Routledge.

Florêncio, João and Ben Miller. 2022. "Sexing the Archive: Gay Porn and Subcultural Histories." *Radical History Review*, 142:133–141.

Foerster, Maxime and Daniel Maroun. 2021. "Introduction: The Show Must Go On: HIV/AIDS and Queer Studies in Twenty-First-Century France." *Contemporary French Civilization*, 46, 2: 121–127.

"Global Statistics." *HIV.gov*. https://www.hiv.gov/hiv-basics/overview/data-and-trends/global-statistics (accessed November 2021)

Greenfeld, Karl Taro. 2020. "The Pattern That Epidemics Always Follow." *The Atlantic*. https://www.theatlantic.com/ideas/archive/2020/03/four-things-you-need-know-about-virus/607495/.

Healy, Patrick. 2014. "A Lion Still Roars, With Gratitude." *New York Times*, May 21. https://www.nytimes.com/2014/05/25/arts/television/larry-kramer-lives-to-see-his-normal-heart-filmed-for-tv.html (accessed 20 December 2021).

Hirsch, Marianne. 2008. "The Generation of Postmemory." *Poetics Today.* Vol. 29, No.1.

Ledin, Chase. 2021. "Retroactivism and Futurity in *120 BPM* and *Théo et Hugo*." *Modern and Contemporary France*. https://doi.org/10.1080/09639489.2021.2000952.

Macron, Emmanuel. 2020. "Adresse aux Français." Speech. Paris. March 16. https://www.elysee.fr/toutes-les-actualites.

Pearl, Monica B. 2012. *AIDS Literature and Gay Identity: The Literature of Loss.* New York: Routledge.

Race, Kane. 2015. "Reluctant Objects: Sexual Pleasure as a Problem for HIV Biomedical Prevention." *GLQ*, Vol. 22, No.1.

Rodríguez, Juana María. 2014. *Sexual Futures, Queer Gestures, and Other Latina Longings*. New York: New York University Press.

Russell, Francey. 2014. "The Unknown Inside." *LA Review of Books*. https://lareviewofbooks.org/article/unknown-inside/.

Schulman, Sarah. 2012. *The Gentrification of the Mind: Witness to a Lost Imagination.* Berkeley, CA: University of California Press.

Shepherd, Jack. 2018. "120 BPM Director Robin Campillo: 'We Were Too Young to Die.'" *Independent*. https://www.independent.co.uk/arts-entertainment/films/features/120-bpm-robin-campillo-interview-act-up-aids-movie-hiv-french-a8290636.html (accessed November 2021)

Shilts, Randy. 1987. *And the Band Played On: Politics, People, and the AIDS Epidemic*. New York: St. Martin's Press.

Tougaw, Jason. 2002. "Testimony and the Subjects of AIDS Memoirs." *Extremities: Trauma, Testimony, and Community.* Edited by Miller, Nancy K. & Tougaw, Jason, University of Illinois Press.

Treichler. Paula A. 1999. *How to Have Theory in an Epidemic*. Durham: Duke University Press.

Watney, Simon. 1987. *Policing Desire: Pornography, AIDS, and the Media*. Minneapolis: University of Minnesota Press.

Woubshet, Dagmawi. 2015. *The Calendar of Loss: Race, Sexuality, and Mourning in the Early Era of AIDS*. Baltimore, MD: Johns Hopkins University Press.

NOTES

1. We agree with Francey Russell who argues in "The Unknown Inside" that "It would not be wrong to see *L'inconnu du lac* as an erotic thriller pivoting on the question of how to live with AIDS—as a person, as a couple, and as a community—some 30 years after it came into our world" (2014).

2. For a thorough examination of the criticism of Lestrade's anti-sex politics, see: Christophe Broqua (2020).

3. This use of intergenerational transmission is in part indebted to Marianne Hirsch's notion of Postmemory. For more, see: Hirsch, Marianne. "The Generation of Postmemory." *Poetics Today.* Vol. 29, No. 1, 2008.

4. For more, see: Pearl, Monica B. *AIDS Literature and Gay Identity: The Literature of Loss.* New York. Routledge, 2012. Schulman, Sarah. *The Gentrification of the Mind: Witness to a Lost Imagination.* University of California Press, 2012. Tougaw, Jason. "Testimony and the Subjects of AIDS Memoirs." *Extremities: Trauma, Testimony, and Community.* Edited by Miller, Nancy K. and Tougaw, Jason, University of Illinois Press, 2002.

5. For an insightful analysis of how PrEP bridges a gap between the HIV-positive and the HIV-negative, see: Caron, David. "Truvada Mon Amour." *The Brooklyn Quarterly*, 13 Nov. 2014.

6. On the political stakes of PrEP, see: Race, Kane. "Reluctant Objects: Sexual Pleasure as a Problem for HIV Biomedical Prevention." *GLQ*, Vol. 22, No. 1, 2015.

Chapter One

Transmitting It

Rawness and the Politics of HIV/AIDS Witnessing Today

David Caron

There is something a little unsettling, for scholars like me who started to write about HIV/AIDS cultural production "back then," in tackling the subject after all these years. Is it even the same subject anyway? The virus is still with us, of course, and numerous communities here and around the world remain perilously vulnerable to it. Old wounds are still raw, what's more, and so are feelings. But by and large, the crisis has abated and, with it, the extraordinary cultural output that characterized the first decade and a half of the known epidemic. Whereas most testimonies, literary or otherwise, used to be produced at the time by people in the process of dying, most witnesses today tend to be activists and other important figures who survived these awful years and now wish to tell their stories. Some, a few, have shared their experience of contracting and living with the virus today, without the fear of impending death, hoping somehow to counter the tidy discourses of closure and erasure that have taken hold in western cultures with regards to HIV. Many, it seems, are demanding some form of reckoning or, to put it more bluntly, justice.[1] I would like to suggest that AIDS writing, today's and yesterday's, may hold a unique power of disruption and that, by extension, when writing on this writing, we should endeavor to bring out and amplify this potential against the forces of cultural denial that have fed the epidemic from the outset and now threaten to rewrite its history.

Cultures forget. In particular, they tend to forget—that is to say, deny—the collective violence they have unleashed in the past, especially upon their own people. At the same time, cultures also tend to selectively remember past misdeeds in order to sustain the narrative of perfectibility on which modern cultures' futurity depends. This, I believe, explains the otherwise baffling success of the movie *Green Book*, the embarrassing winner of the Best Picture Oscar for 2018. We are authorized—indeed exhorted—to revisit the history of segregation and celebrate how far we have come as a nation, how we no longer commit such blatant acts of racial injustice. Except, of course, that we do. But denial is precisely the point. Sanctioned memory demands that troubling facts be transformed, processed, either by radically othering the past ("Vichy wasn't France") or by attenuating the seriousness of the crimes ("Colonialism benefitted to the colonized"). Personal testimonies of historical acts of violence, however, may offer stubborn resistance to this kind of oblivion and denial. Still, whether witnesses succeed in offering counter-narratives to dominant cultural forces depends on how their accounts are received and what those who receive them do with these testimonies. What, then, in the era of effective treatments and prophylaxis, is the point of testifying to one's own experience of living with HIV? What is at play in testimonies from the early years and by those who survived them? Does HIV/AIDS still offer us anything relevant to make politics with? Following the works of scholars who consider the reception of witnessing practices to be a witnessing practice in its own right, I wonder what ethical and political demands HIV/AIDS witnessing makes of its recipients today.

THE RAW AND THE COOKED

The question of rawness that grounds this volume provides us with a critical tool with which to begin to sort out this recent cultural production and to lay its stakes bare, so to speak. For academics, the word raw may first bring to mind Claude Lévi-Strauss's essay *The Raw and the Cooked*. Lévi-Strauss, as we know, does not have much to say about rawness in particular. The book's title announces its focus on structural dichotomies rooted in the sensory experience of everyday life, of which the raw and the cooked is one among many, but which serve as a basis for abstract conceptualization—food for thought, really, and not a bad place to start reflecting on raw writing. Indeed, to call writing raw automatically presupposes the existence or possibility of writing that *isn't* raw and that, therefore, must be cooked or otherwise processed. Clearly, "cooked," as an adjective, has not spawned the sort of metaphorical progeny that "raw" has, so we must turn instead to those metaphors for fruitful opposites.

In the context of HIV/AIDS, "raw" immediately evokes unprotected anal sex. The practice known as "barebacking" made its first controversial splash in the late 1990s, when HIV-positive LGBT+ activist Tony Valenzuela went public about his preference for condomless sex, a taste that gay men broadly shared and increasingly practiced but seldom discussed openly for fear of social or legal consequences. Social critics, such as Kane Race, Gregory Tomso, and Tim Dean, soon went on to observe and theorize raw sex and bring out its potential for culture-making, political critique, transgression, or the reimagining of kinship for queer purposes. Sometimes, they reminded us that sex without condoms just feels better. Today, with effective treatments and the use of pre-exposure prophylaxis, or PrEP, unprotected sex has become too common to retain its critical edge as an actual practice. By extension, to prefer to have protected sex cannot fairly be taken as a sign of reactionary politics.

Given this intellectual and social history, extending the concept of rawness to writing represents a political move. It inevitably hints at a metaphorical risk of infection with something we'd be wise to avoid but also at a desire for unmediated queer intimacy—perhaps both at once sometimes. Either way, to speak of raw writing, in that sense, can only imply consequences for its recipients, be they individual readers or the culture at large. Metaphors of risky, unprotected reading as a challenge to ontological, social, or political homogeneity featured prominently in early queer theorizing of AIDS cultural production as a combat weapon. Infection could be reclaimed figuratively against the dominant discourses that made the epidemic possible in the first place, threatening entire communities with extinction. In today's post-crisis reality, however, this approach has largely fallen into disuse. HIV sucks and it is scary but it does not really transgress anything anymore. And as of this writing, it is too soon to know if, in the aftermath of the seemingly never-ending COVID-19 crisis, the metaphor of infection will once more come to advocate for contact in a world increasingly promoting distancing, social and otherwise. I doubt it, though.

But raw writing need not be limited to transgression and metaphorical infection in order to retain some political force. Form, literary or otherwise figurative, is contact surface and thus relational by definition. Formal choices thus perform modes of relationality. In the specific context of French AIDS literature, for example, commentators often pair and oppose Hervé Guibert and Guillaume Dustan, admittedly the two best and most important authors in the AIDS genre, or whatever it is. Guibert, while young, was *Le Monde*'s photography critic and already had many books under his belt when his 1990 testimonial volume on living with AIDS, *A l'ami qui ne m'a pas sauvé la vie* (1990) [*To the Friend Who Did Not Save My Life* (1991)], became a huge critical and commercial success. Dustan, on the other hand, was a complete newcomer whose 1996 *Dans ma chambre* [*In My Room* (1998)] dragged the question of barebacking into the open and ignited a heated controversy among a narrower audience of gay readers. It was not long before a simplistic view of the differences between the two authors took hold: on one side a polished writer, friends with Michel Foucault and Isabelle Adjani, published by Gallimard and feted by the media; on the other an initially unseen nobody writing under a pseudonym in community-based gay slang and quasi-pornographic style about taking giant dildos up the ass. In reality, Dustan's writing was in its own way just as literate and rigorously crafted as Guibert's, whom he acknowledged as a model of AIDS autofiction. And even the contrast between the apparent consensus that greeted Guibert's crossover success and the mix of admiration and condemnation facing a lesser-known Dustan should not hide the fact that Dustan, too, became an established writer in his own right, and one who, like Guibert, has become the subject of rereleases, biographies and academic studies.

As for the question of raw writing as risky, Guibert, the supposedly "safer" author, directly goads readers into contemplating the possibility of infection through reading, as when he describes the influence of Austrian writer Thomas Bernhard on his own writing as an act that recalls HIV transmission:

> parallèlement donc au virus VIH la métastase bernhardienne s'est propagée à la vitesse grand V dans mes tissus et mes réflexes vitaux d'écriture, elle . . . en détruit tout naturel et toute personnalité . . . j'attends avec impatience le vaccin littéraire qui me délivrera du sortilège que je me suis infligé à dessein par l'entremise de Thomas Bernhard, transformant l'observation et l'admiration de son écriture . . . en menace pathogène, en sida. (1990, 216–17)
>
> [this Bernhardian metastasis has spread just like the HIV virus at Top Speed . . . through the viral tissues and reflexes of my writing . . . destroying all its personality and natural qualities . . . I impatiently await the literary vaccine that will deliver me from the spell I purposefully cast upon myself through Thomas Bernhard, transforming the observation and admiration of his writing . . . into a pathogenic threat, into AIDS" (1991, 198–99)]

Far from being a tame and tidy witness, Guibert shrinks the safe distance between him and his readers and invites them to shatter their sense of self in a way made comparable to his own undoing by HIV. His explicit self-referentiality and implicit calls to readers make his writing writerly, as Barthes defines the term in *Le plaisir du texte* (1973) [*The Pleasure of the Text*]: sexualized, unruly, and ontologically dangerous. If Guibert's attacks on safe reading do not seem as belligerent today as they did at first, it may simply be because we are now reading him after the crisis. But just as we find that the disruptive power of Holocaust witness literature has not abated decades after the liberation of the camps, we can still turn to Guibert's AIDS autofiction for a profound critique of modern, bourgeois concepts of the self and the subject.

In addition to its connotations of sex and risk, the word *raw* also evokes something direct and honest, realer, the opposite of artificial or fake, especially when applied to expressions of emotions or depictions of the world. To communicate in such unadulterated fashion, albeit within socially sanctioned limits, is supposed to signal authenticity, both in art and in our relations with others and the world. Again, we may be tempted to interpret Guibert's elegant literariness as more conventional and less queer than Dustan's provocative obscenities. But this again simplifies the question, as we can see when looking side by side at two passages I chose (almost) randomly as representative of the two authors' respective stylistic approach to descriptions of gay sex. Each depicts a three-way and raises the issues of orgasm, risk, and ambivalent reluctance in transgressive terms:

> J'avais toujours pris des précautions avec le Poète, même lorsqu'il m'avait prié de le traiter comme une chienne, et que je l'avais livré à Jules, me servant de Jules comme d'un godemiché que je ne souhaitais pas être. J'avais senti juste avant la jouissance une très étrange sueur monter de nos trois corps imbriqués, c'était la plus voluptueuse des odeurs, la plus vertigineuse aussi: je me demandai si nous n'étions pas devenus, Jules et moi, un couple d'assassins sauvages sans foi ni loi. (Guibert 1990, 160)
>
> [I'd always taken precautions with the Poet, even when he'd begged me to treat him like a slut, and when I'd handed him over to Jules, whom I used as the dildo I didn't care to be. Just before orgasm, I'd smelled a very strange sweat emanating from our overlapping bodies, the most voluptuous of odors, and the most staggering: I wondered if Jules and I hadn't become a pair of savages, godless murderers. (1991, 144)]

And:

> Une fois j'ai partouzé comme ça avec deux mecs, moi j'ai calé, je débandais dans leur cul et quand ils me sautaient, ça me faisait trop flipper de baiser à risques, ok on ne sait rien sur la réinfection mais ce qui est sûr c'est qu'en faisant ce genre de choses on peut se choper des tas de trucs en plus. Cela dit, quand le petit vicelard a giclé sans capote dans le cul du grand skin, c'était vertigineux. Le baiser de la mort, comme on dit. (Dustan 1996, 133)
>
> [One time in a three-way I kept losing my hard-on in their asses, and when they fucked me I was too freaked out having unsafe sex. OK, we don't know anything about reinfection but we do know that with this kind of thing we can catch a lot more crap. Even so, when the little nasty guy with no condom shot off in the tall skinhead's ass it was breathtaking. The kiss of death they say (1998, 104).]

Beyond the similarities in the acts they depict, the two excerpts resemble each other in how they represent raw sex as disturbingly seductive. In the end, both authors use the same adjective, *vertigineux*, to describe what they're feeling. (The English translations opt for "staggering" with Guibert and "breathtaking" with Dustan.) Granted, Dustan writes in a quasi-spoken style and uses technical slang for this act or that, while Guibert writes more classically. But how significant is this stylistic difference if ultimately both passages seek to induce in their readers the same disquieting mixture of pleasure and repulsion they are themselves experimenting?

Yes, there is something undeniably fresh and exciting about Dustan's writing, but Guibert's is not exactly tame stuff either. To be blunt, they both made me hard when I first read them. And in keeping with erotic literary tradition, they both conjure up the age-old appeal of the dizzying dance of Eros and Thanatos. How then should we account for the differences between them? Guibert, as signaled by his recognizable literariness and *parisiannisme*, belongs to a certain French literary tradition of dark eroticism that links Sade, Bataille, Genet, Catherine Millet, and others. And while Dustan is also guilty of *parisianisme* and explicitly positions himself as heir to this history, he hijacks it and takes it to its next phase, one that represents both a break and a continuation and would include, for example, a major figure like Virginie Despentes. But Guibert and Dustan overlap in significant ways in their use of autofiction and, of course, by writing primarily not about sex but about AIDS, making Guibert a bridge figure in literary history. Whether rawness separates or unites Guibert and Dustan makes little difference in the end. Each wrote obscenely and each, as witness to the catastrophe of AIDS, showed deep concern with the question of form in relation to HIV literary transmission.

As I see it, the problem lies not in the differences between the two authors but in the internal contradiction that immediately arises when we define rawness as authenticity. Paradoxical as it may sound, the social valuation given authenticity in post-Romantic cultures exposes the notion, and with it all desire for naturalness, as an artifice. In our interactions, we get off on the *idea* of authenticity and on the value we attribute to it more often than on authenticity itself, which, like "nature," would remain conceptually inaccessible without some sort of discursive mediation in any case. As an ideal, there is no such thing as raw rawness. Not to mention the fact that the ideal of purity that inheres in the association of raw with authentic all but negates rawness's supposed openness to (contamination by) others. In short, if rawness as form invites relationality, it calls for its own refashioning by others and must therefore forgo all claims to original authenticity.

While I prefer to turn away from uses of rawness as infection and authenticity—the first because it is critically outdated, the second because it is a logical impossibility—I find that they do share a helpful premise: the opposition between the raw and the *no longer* raw inevitably implies temporality. Rawness, in that sense, suggests an initial state, something like the primal stage in a process of change. To fuck without a condom, say, means to return to sex as it was before AIDS, to sex as it was meant to be. And the yearning for authenticity fuels a larger project of self-actualization often understood as ridding oneself of the suffocating layers of civilization and returning to modes of existence perceived as older, simpler, truer. Think of Michel, the protagonist of Gide's *L'immoraliste* (1902) [*The Immoralist* (1930)], for whom absence of civilization signifies freedom. Raw, in that sense, takes on the two meanings of the French *cru*: raw but also crude. Raw comes before, whether or not anything actually follows it.

"Crude," however, raises the same objections as "authentic." Both are cultural, not elemental, and thus self-contradictory. In terms of temporality, an early stage can only be called that from the perspective of future developments. Similarly, something may be described as crude insofar as improvements have subsequently occurred or are felt to be needed. To value crudeness as such, then, inevitably entails a reimagining of the past, which was at the time neither crude nor the past. Crude writing valued as crude is thus always rewriting, as we can see if we turn to the early French witness literature of AIDS for an example.

Michel Simonin, whom Jean-Pierre Boulé once called "a forgotten witness" (2002, 90), belongs to a small group of French people with AIDS who wrote about their experience during the early years of the epidemic. To be exact, I should say that they wrote about their experience during the early years of AIDS witness literature in France. The success of Guibert's *A l'ami* didn't trigger this literature so much as public interest for it. As many authors appeared on the scene and the epidemic became so bad it could no longer be ignored, earlier witnesses died and their work vanished with them. One of them was Simonin. I stumbled upon his 1986 memoir *Danger de vie* [*Danger of Life*] in a gay bookstore in Montreal years after its release. I had never heard of Simonin and could not wait to read his book. The story provided a candid and revealing account of the life of a gay man with AIDS in the mid-1980s. It was honest, it was blunt, it was raw, and it was awful.

At a time when I was devoting much of my work to Guibert and others, I could not help but wonder what it was exactly that made this particular book practically unreadable. It would be telling to contrast excerpts from Simonin's account of his daily life in the hospital with some taken from Guibert's own hospital diary, *Cytomégalovirus* (1992) [*Cytomegalovirus: A Hospitalization Diary* (2016)]. Whereas the later author penned a barebones, harrowing screed against dehumanizing institutional power ("Rien écrit ce soir. Trop choqué. J'essaierai demain" (59) [Wrote nothing this evening. Too shell-shocked. I'll try tomorrow. (56)]), the other devotes pages and pages to reviewing the television programs he watches all day long. One text uses rawness as art; the other simply leaves experience unprocessed. *Danger de vie* has genuine value as a historical document but quoting it to make my point would be facile and cruel. Simonin deserves respect for his courage. We should honor him for his willingness to testify at a time when people with AIDS were met with indifference or hatred and no community supported them. But this case of unadorned self-expression, while personally vital in the face of the radical loss of self that is AIDS, nonetheless exemplifies what happens to writing that is not "raw" but raw: it is unreadable because neglectful of its afterlife. If, as I wrote, raw always comes before, raw writing as a political practice exists for the effects it seeks to produce. Its purpose is not to reclaim some authenticity supposedly found in earlier forms but, rather, to use the unsettling interplay of past, present, and future to propose a radical concept of witness temporality.

Referring to the history of AIDS, I described feelings and old wounds as raw, or to be exact, *still* raw. In these common phrases, raw signifies that some sort of metaphorical healing has not taken place as it was expected to. Wounds and feelings are not supposed to remain raw; as the culture around us never ceases to remind us, we are supposed to strive for closure and move on. In our context, though, we may understand healing in its literal sense as well, a reminder that there still exists no cure for HIV, no vaccine against it, and that the AIDS pandemic is still ongoing. We could then envision uses of rawness as an active rebuttal to the sort of closure sought not by the people most affected by HIV/AIDS but by those bent on denial. Either way and to the extent that, as per Levi-Strauss, the word could not exist without its opposite, raw is not just raw; it means not yet processed, it means unfinished. Raw has a future. Raw represents a stubbornly, irritatingly extended present of suffering that aspires to its own end ("J'essaierai demain" ["I'll try tomorrow"]) but demands to have a say in making the future. We may then reconcile trope and denotation and critically use the concept of rawness to keep calling for an end to the pandemic and also to demand that justice be done for those it has killed or otherwise touched.

Finally, the phrase "raw writing" itself contains two possible opposites: cooked writing and raw reading. The first opposite suggests a kind of cultural product that would adhere too closely to codes and conventions to yield any meaningful surprises and qualify as art; all *techne* and no *poiesis*. In that sense, the phrase echoes the difference French film critic Serge Daney posited between raw and cooked cinema, the latter having had all life and urgency processed out of it. He hastens to specify, however, that the two cannot be so neatly distinguished: "Entre le document et le fictif, le brut et le codé, les aléas et le dispositif, bref entre *le cru et le cuit*, il y a toujours eu court-circuit, raccourci saisissant, impureté" ["Between document and fiction, the crude and the coded, vagaries and apparatus, in short between *the raw and the cooked*, there has always been short-circuits, striking shortcuts, impurity" (my translation).] (*La rampe*, 195; original emphasis). In a later interview, however, Daney made it clear that by "cooked" cinema he means conventional films similar to the ones François Truffaut attacked as a young critic—bourgeois cinema.[2]

The second opposite, raw reading, may puzzle at first blush. To be sure, how can reading be unprocessed given the delay and distance that characterize the act of reading in the first place? To read *is* to process. By the same token, this could just as well be said of writing in relation to reality. Putting this technical objection aside, what I find promising in the concept of raw reading is that it shifts the emphasis to reception, that is, to the future, already present in rawness but also in writing as founding absence and possibility. Both "raw" and "writing" always already contain (the necessity of) something yet to come. Raw is raw to the strict extent that it may be cooked later; writing is writing in that it necessarily posits an addressee, if only as an implied reader. This is basic deconstruction, of course, but what sounds like an abstract disruption of temporality opens up the possibility of actual practices. Can raw reading, whatever that may look like concretely, provide a way for rawness to have a future without relinquishing the stubborn, disturbing presentness that gives it its critical force?

WHAT WITNESSING DOES

This notion that life may all at once be itself and its own aftermath has a name: it is called survival; life that goes on in excess of itself, after it was supposed to have ended. Survival, needless to say, lies at the core of the literature of AIDS, alongside other forms of witness literature that demands of its readers that they keep the wound and the feelings raw until the dead and the survivors receive the justice that they are owed. Raw writing, in that sense, would be the sort of writing that demands that its unsettling incompletion be prolonged into the reading so that readers may in turn continue to convey it and, as I would like to argue, envision not simply justice for a specific group but a just world. In other words, if reading is the future of witness writing, justice is the future of witness reading.

In *Facing It*, Ross Chambers seeks to resolve a tension between engagement and concern as possible reactions to reading AIDS witness literature. Looking at Eric Michaels' memoir *Unbecoming*, Chambers defines the terms as follows. Concern "is a way of disengaging oneself and one's responsibility, but without seeming to, according to a duplicitous structure that would align concern with tidiness" (1998, 110); concern is bourgeois, whereas engagement, which authors such as Michaels demand from their audience, throws the readers into a situation they cannot control, thus putting these readers' self at risk and at stake. Engagement disempowers, it is messy and untidy; it is anti-bourgeois. The duplicity and distancing that define concern come in sharp contrast with the rawness of engagement. But true, raw engagement via reading remains inevitably out of reach because of who actually makes up the reading public of AIDS literature and because reading, as I recalled, presupposes remoteness. If engagement cannot but fail and if concern is the only remaining yet unacceptable choice, then, Chambers concludes, anxious reading may bring a way out of the readers' conundrum: "Engaged reading, then, in its ideal form, is a utopia. The best a militantly uncompliant text . . . can achieve, although it is somewhat less than it demands, is [a] sort of anxiously involved reading . . . a reading that is uncertain of itself because it is conscious, however hard it tries, of its own failure to be anything but concerned" (113). When success is not an option, what matters is how to fail right.

If anxiety signals that one's reading has failed successfully, as it were, excessive empathy represents the sort of success that fails outright. There is nothing inherently wrong with empathy, but what I call excessive empathy is the sort that ultimately denies the witnesses' otherness by dispossessing them of their stories. Working from testimonies of the Holocaust and Nazi concentration camps, Thomas Trezise insists that whoever receives these stories must empathize without identifying with the witnesses. Only by embracing the inevitable discomfort that comes with our inability to empathize in full can we in turn become the witnesses of these witnesses. As he writes, "the witnesses of witnessing are required to maintain a balance of empathy and reserve, to tolerate a tension between identification and estrangement, to recognize and respect the irreducible otherness of survivors while, in effect, welcoming them back into the larger community" (2013, 224). As we saw with Chambers, the "bad" feelings we experience when engaging with the words of witnesses bespeak our inevitable shortcomings and failure to meet the demands they place on us. The readers' challenge, I would add, is to accept incongruence—in psychological terms, the discrepancy between our feelings and our actions—as, if not the most desirable, the least undesirable outcome.

Continuing this conversation in *On the Defensive*, Sharon Marquart questions the very ethical impulses that move us toward witness literature in the first place. Even the most well-intentioned of readers, she warns, risk erasing the witnesses' irreducible otherness. In this case, denial does not issue from duplicity or an avowed desire to tidy up a messy world at other people's expense, but from a tendency to inscribe one's reception within a culturally shared system of ethics that validates that reception as appropriate but also "den[ies] the disturbance of testimony" (2015, 5). In other words, if we want to do justice to witnesses, we must jettison the very notion of ethics that triggers our desire to hear them in the first place. If witnesses are to be welcomed back into a community, the demand is on us to resist using ethics as a pre-established code or apparatus, to recall Daney's terms, that would remain somehow unaffected by the untidiness that survivors and other witnesses bring with them into the world.

If receiving witness literature constitutes that literature's afterlife, the way to do it justice is to relay and perpetuate the disturbance it conveys, to keep the wound and the feelings raw, even though reception is always a mode of processing things. The best way to resolve this particular incongruence—raw and cooked at the same time—is to embrace another one, one which defines survival—the coexistence of life and no-longer-life.

Witness writing, especially of historical catastrophes such as the AIDS pandemic, is collective in nature. Survivors and temporary survivors speak for those who have already died and also for those who have survived but cannot write, i.e., those who cannot process an experience of suffering that must nonetheless be passed on. The self-erasure, or self-dissolution, that characterizes witness writing, but first of all the very experience of catastrophic events, must be somehow experienced not just by those who take in the stories afterward but, if there is to be justice, by the entire culture in which we read. In critical terms, haunting aptly describes this phenomenon.

For Chambers, witness writing is not just haunted, it also haunts, making it what he terms "aftermath writing." Expanding in *Untimely Interventions* the reach of an idea he touched on in *Facing It*, Chambers sees the ongoing transmission of hauntedness from the dead to the living, writers to readers, texts to culture, as a means to foreclose, or at least impede the possibility of denial and tidy distancing—stances cultures tend to adopt with a past that could threaten their existence. Haunting, characterized by temporal disruption—what Chambers calls "untimeliness"—thus comes to figure *cultural* disruption as well:

> Because trauma repeats and returns when it is supposedly over, aftermath writing as a hauntedness that haunts has a double character of untimeliness. It is both an exploration of survival as the experience of untimeliness—that is, of a baffling experience of times as, conjointly, the separation of past and present and their continuing copresence . . . —and an art of untimely intervention, seeking to introduce an awareness of untimeliness into a culture that prefers to live in time as if the past had no place in the present and did not haunt (i.e., inhabit) it. (2004, 191)

In a similar vein, Trezise notes "the in-finitude or nonfiniteness of testimonial interlocution" (2013, 211). I would add that if rawness (understood as the continued suppuration of infected wounds that refuse to heal for someone else's comfort) and crudeness (meaning the dogged inappropriateness of those who will not assimilate to bourgeois norms) manifest their own form of untimeliness, then they too function in the mode of haunting in order to resist the temptation of closure and finitude. Rawness and crudeness usher ghosts into our consciousness and into the culture, ghosts that demand justice, not just for themselves but, through themselves, for the world.

Trezise talked about "welcoming [survivors] back into the larger community." But if we are to do justice to witnesses then community cannot remain untouched by those it welcomes back. Welcoming *back* may in fact not be the right phrase. No matter how you understand the term, community (being relational by definition) keeps being made and remade by those who are in it or constitutionally kept out of it—not to mention continually unmade, like everything else, by time itself. It is thus logically impossible to join the community we aspire to belong to because it ceases to be that community the moment we join it. But for survivors, to rejoin a community as it existed before the events they are testifying to would mean acquiescing to the denial of injustice. What survivors bring with them, then, is a heightened commitment to a just world. Or as Trezise puts it, "the way in which we receive the testimony of Holocaust survivors is inseparable from the way in which we practice, with one another, a present and future community" (226). Marquart goes one step further by suggesting that it may be for us to join the witnesses' community rather than the other way round, as survivors are "working to include us in the communities they construct, and showing us ways to open ourselves up so we can be there for others" (2015, 5). Either way, if rawness conveys a demand for justice, it cannot demand it only for those affected by HIV/AIDS. Rather, it must harness HIV's unique power to expose systemic injustice broadly and, from that perspective, contribute to the collective struggle.

AIDS REDUX

The question of community distinguishes several recent movies about the early years of the AIDS crisis. This particular focus may owe to the collective nature of the film-viewing experience, of course, although streaming is fast changing our habits. More likely, I would like to argue, community acts as a locus for a struggle over competing political visions, one of which consists of a desire to counter the individualization of the illness after 1996 and to reclaim AIDS activism as a possible inspiration for contemporary struggles rooted in group discrimination or global emergencies.[3]

The second decade of the 21st century, the fourth of the known epidemic, has seen a spectacular resurgence of interest in the early years of the AIDS crisis. Important AIDS plays have been revived, among them William Finn's *Falsettos*, William M. Hoffman's *As Is*, Jonathan Larsen's *Rent*, Larry Kramer's *The Normal Heart* and works by Jean-Luc Lagarce. Two documentaries on ACT UP-New York hit the theaters back to back: Jim Hubbard's *United in Anger: A History of ACT UP* and David France's *How to Survive a Plague*. In France, two feature films came out just months apart, both set in the early to mid-1990s, the darkest years: Christophe Honoré's *Plaire, aimer et courir vite* [*Sorry Angel*] (2018) and Robin Campillo's *120 battements par minute* [*BPM*] (2017). Scholars, museum curators, and biographers have started taking fresh looks at artists who died of AIDS, such as David Wojnanowicz and Robert Mapplethorpe. Importantly, surviving activists started publishing personal accounts of their struggles in the early years. Among the most notable in France are a number of autobiographical volumes by ACT UP-Paris cofounder Didier Lestrade and a volume of interview with AIDES founder Daniel Defert, while on this side of the Atlantic, Sean Strub, who started *Poz* magazine, comes to mind. As of this writing, new witness narratives of the period are slated for release from TAG founding members Peter Staley and Mark Harrington, playwright and activist Sarah Schulman, and various other members of ACT UP-New York.[4]

One could propose several explanations for this burst of activity and why it is taking place now. Time passes and becomes history, for one thing, and history must be recorded. Understandably, early activists and other witnesses of the period, whose very lives depended on the production of counter-discourses, intend to play their part in the historiography of a period they helped shape. But another crucial factor, I believe, is the victory in the fight for marriage equality, which many see as the culmination of decades of rights-oriented gay and lesbian activism. This official confirmation of full citizenship, I want to suggest, propelled the need to recover (but really produce) the narrative of progress that at long last brought us here, our final destination. In France as well as in the United States, the AIDS crisis has now largely been inscribed in prevalent cultural narratives as a tragic and, in hindsight, heroic stage on the path to LGBT+ integration and the country's betterment as a civil society.

It could be that the issue of marriage equality found itself at the forefront of gay politics simply because legalization felt like the next logical step in a longer journey toward social justice in general. In France, for example, the seemingly inexorable path from the PaCS [civil partnership] to the *mariage pour tous* [marriage for all] certainly gives the impression that same-sex marriage was indeed an idea whose time had come. Without going over the finer details of how this came to be, it is worth remembering that earlier attempts at legalizing same-sex unions in the form of domestic partnerships did not necessarily appeal to the universal principle of equality but, more often than not, anchored their rhetoric to pragmatic, everyday life concerns expected to resonate more convincingly with the public at large. Featured prominently were the tragic situations that arose from the AIDS crisis: lovers with no hospital visitation rights; friends who provided care from the start sidelined at the last minute by greedy, homophobic relatives nobody even knew; life partners expelled from their apartments because the lease could only be in the name of one person, now dead. The inhumane treatment of people with AIDS and of the friends who cared physically and materially for them occupied a central part in the legalization rhetoric and contributed its fair share to rallying a sympathetic public to the cause.

By the time same-sex marriage became law, however, this was no longer the case, as the cause sought support primarily by relying on the rhetoric of equality as a universal aspiration rather than as an answer to people's concrete needs. Visitation rights and other administrative entitlements hadn't vanished from this rhetoric; what had vanished, or at least faded, is the issue's link to HIV and AIDS. In our liberal-democratic society, the purpose of equality, it seems, is no longer the just treatment of vulnerable flesh-and-blood human beings but open access to goods and services. I do not mean to sound dismissive. In fact, one could argue that the amazing progress in the treatment of HIV which, for many, has transformed the disease into a manageable chronic condition, explains why hospital visitation rights seem self-evident whether you are gay or not. If we no longer bring up the tragedies of the past, that is precisely because they are of the past. They have done their job, as it were, and they will not help when homophobic florists and cake makers try to ruin the party you are entitled to as a consumer.

Two recent French memoirs illustrate this turn in post-marriage HIV/AIDS cultural production. One, Camille Genton's *Positif* [*Positive*] (2017), tells the story of a 25-year-old gay entrepreneur who unexpectedly receives an HIV-positive diagnosis as he is about to settle down with his boyfriend. Once the shock recedes and the treatment successfully reduces his viral load to undetectable levels, Camille goes on with his life opening restaurants in Paris, only to find his business ambitions hampered by outdated regulations that make bank loans inaccessible to people with HIV and other long-term illnesses. He then makes it his mission to have the rules rescinded, and that is when the reader realizes that the entire book has been a platform for Genton's cause and that the title referred not just to the author's HIV status but to his liberal credo of self-accomplishment.[5]

Less openly Macronist[6] but just about as captivating is Lucie Hovhannessian's *Presque comme les autres* [*Almost Like Everyone Else*] (2018), in which we learn that young, heterosexual Lucie fears being considered a dumb slut for having so carelessly contracted HIV. Thankfully (for her), she gets over these negative feelings, drops out of college, and keeps on enjoying sex with boys, Rihanna concerts, and a thoroughly ordinary life, the details of which she relates in the most tedious manner as HIV becomes as undetectable in the book as it is in her bloodstream.[7] In a sense, these two memoirs find their place alongside, not earlier works of AIDS witness literature, but sundry other books relating how someone has managed to overcome a serious ordeal of one kind or another and reclaim some normalcy in their life. Normalcy, as Hovhannessian's title suggests, is indeed the purpose of these two books. HIV must no longer stand in the way of enjoying the benefits that a liberal society is meant to provide to every individual citizen/consumer. That, apparently, is what we fought for all along.

But from a new generation of academics and activists comes a different, not so tidy story, one that does not look into history for a backstory to the triumph of assimilationist LGBT+ politics but, on the contrary, mines the past for inspiration to fuel new forms of activism more focused on systemic change than on individual rights. For many younger people who have also manifested a keen interest in the epidemic's early years, the AIDS crisis does not represent a historical tragedy so much as a precursor to current social movements inscribed within a larger fight for a global politics of justice. With that in mind, the question that arises is whether we can, today, write about HIV/AIDS in the (singular or plural) first-person testimonial mode without being coopted into a liberal version of our own history. Can HIV/AIDS testimonial writing, and artistic practices in general, contribute to the fight for global justice rather than feed the heroic narrative of rights and legal equality that depends on forgetting and denial? Ultimately at stake, both in memory work and in new cultural productions, is whether AIDS will be relegated to the safe confines of the past or continue to haunt us, to remain with us as a tenacious irritant and a counterforce to liberal ideals predicated on forgetting their complicity in mass death.

The two documentaries about ACT UP-New York, *How to Survive a Plague* and *United in Anger* offer a telling contrast. The first presents us with a heroic narrative of reconciliation that, by celebrating heroes once repelled as diseased outcasts and poisoners of wells, makes us all heroes for embracing them. *United in Anger* looks more like a manual for activism. One movie gets nominated for an Oscar and pops up often on syllabi and campus events; the other was screened but not distributed and may be facing oblivion thanks to the usual gatekeepers.[8] Both movies make ample use of ACT UP's visual archive documenting the spectacular actions the group was famous for. But *How to Survive a Plague* soon veers in a different direction and begins to tell the story of a small band of activists who left ACT UP to create the Treatment Action Group (TAG) and focus their efforts on medical research rather than politics. As the focus of the movie changes, so does its portrayal of AIDS activism. From the messy and confrontational tactics of ACT UP emerges a more pragmatic and, according to the movie, more effective approach based on dialogue and collaboration with medical institutions. TAG members become the true heroes of the story as they mature away from their rambunctious beginnings and transform into responsible advocates. In a classic narrative arc, injustice begets disorder, but only with order restored shall justice prevail in the end. Already conventional in form, with its linear chronology, sense of closure and familiar blend of archival footage and talking heads, the movie also resorts to a rather manipulative narrative artifice. For a while, TAG members only appear onscreen in images from the period, and as viewers are made to feel increasingly attached to them, worries increase as well. Are these guys still alive or did they not make it? As their one-by-one appearance as talking heads soon reveal, they did survive after all, and along with our relief comes a sense that these heroes have been duly rewarded for their work and their courage. The title of the movie now becomes clear: in order to survive a plague, that is, in order to appear in its historiography, you must fit in the narrative of futurity and crisis resolution that this historiography propels. In the end, *How to Survive a Plague* may owe its recognition to its stealthy dequeering of ACT UP and its tidy mode of (not) witnessing.

If raw history must be processed for easier digestion, *United in Anger* will keep you up at night. Messy, unruly, and as crude in form as it is raw in affects, this movie remains firmly planted in ACT UP itself and in its queer collective ethos. As a result, it creates a sense of unfinished business radically at odds with a vision of futurity premised on selective oblivion and the restoration of order. Narratively untidy, the movie turns away from the confining structure of generic forms, intensifying a feeling of continued urgency that capitalizes on ACT UP's energy and makes you want to get in on the action. Although not necessarily for the specific purpose of fighting AIDS, which today would look nothing like it did then. *United in Anger* does not bring closure to history; it breaches its boundaries and makes the kind of activism that ACT UP pioneered feel irrepressibly alive and pertinent no matter the cause. It could just as well be Black Lives Matter or #MeToo or Extinction Rebellion. Paradoxically, it is by not emphasizing survival that the movie feels so alive today. The unity and anger of the title, embodied by so many vibrant human beings now almost all dead, are passed on to us. Rather than mourn their loss, we become haunted by their raging spirit. At a campus screening followed by a Q&A with the director, I heard students ask, "Why weren't we told about this?" The movie constructs a community you want to join. Unlike the reassuring sense of closure that *How to Survive a Plague* aims to provide, *United in Anger* makes community attractive in the full sense of the word: it is sexy, it is open, and we want in.

A similar energy permeates the French feature film *120 battements par minute* [*BPM*]. This movie, written and directed by Robin Campillo based on his own experience with ACT UP-Paris and fictionalizing real events and real people, was met with near unanimous praise. It won numerous awards, including the Grand Prix at the Cannes film festival and the César for best film of 2017, and became a cultural phenomenon of sorts. The story is set in the mid-1990s and follows two main characters, Sean and Nathan, as they go through their lives as AIDS activists and face Sean's deteriorating health and eventual death. The focus on the lovers feels like a small concession to cinematic narrative conventions, however, given that the movie foregrounds the daily life of ACT UP itself so as to make the group not a mere background for the characters but the central topic. An unusually high amount of screen time is devoted to contentious weekly meetings, and we see a fairly accurate array of ACT UP's spectacular public actions, always filmed from the activists' point of view, the camera moving with and within the group. The effect is to systematically shift the narrative from the personal to the collective, from the self-actualizing to the selfless.

Campillo especially favors this approach when presenting the death of a beloved character and thus the literal selflessness that awaited so many AIDS activists at the time. One of these characters in the movie is Jérémie, a sweet, lovely young man whose health soon takes a turn for the worse. The movie does not show us his death, though, and cuts directly to what ACT UP called a political funeral: turning the death of one of them into a public event. In this case, activists follow the hearse carrying Jérémie's casket on the street holding a bunch of placards with his portrait on them and the caption "Jérémie est mort du sida" [Jérémie died of AIDS] (*BPM*, 2017). Again, the camera is located amid the marchers. These multiple images of the young man's face, with the cause of death reclaimed in a public space, dilute his singularity and turn him into an emblem to be followed not in death but in action. As for Sean's death at the end of the movie, it is tougher to take for viewers, who for the past two hours have fallen under the spell of his vital energy and charisma. But a political funeral follows when the activists break into a buffet reception by an insurance company and scatter his ashes all over the place. This radical, posthumous action by the now selfless Sean matches our heightened sense of loss and anger at the death of the beloved protagonist, but his dissemination as ashes also pulverizes his potential heroism. Sean has turned into an angry ghost. This scene ends the movie but does not close it any more than Sean's death has ended his activism with ACT UP. By echoing the opening episode, an action during which an activist throws fake blood at a government official, the movie moves from fake blood to real ashes and creates a cyclical rather than linear structure that creates momentum and resonates as a call for continued action.

Sure enough, and this may be the most unexpected outcome of *BPM*'s popularity among young gay men (which I have witnessed among my own students when I teach it), the movie generated so much excitement that an almost moribund ACT UP-Paris saw a sudden surge in membership. The new members, however, quickly overthrew the group's leadership which they found too narrowly focused on HIV at this post-crisis stage in the epidemic's history. Instead, they pushed for a new agenda more in tune with the organization's founding spirit, which understood the spread of HIV/AIDS as resulting from a systemic aggregate of interrelated oppressions. AIDS activism may never again look like what we see in *United in Anger* and *BPM*, and we should rejoice at the thought, but it should not be forgotten or entirely abandoned either. With these movies, something of its raw appeal allows that pandemic to live on and haunt today's global radical politics, fueling the sense of geographic and historical interconnectedness that propels it.

Illness memoirs and documentary films, when they are intelligent, can have a lot to say about what it means to be human and facing bodily decay, fragility, loss of autonomy, impairment, death. But testifying about AIDS was never about illness; it was about injustice. Even when you testify in a court of law, it is about justice. The best works of witness emerging from the crisis testify to that. As they stubbornly resist their appropriation into a narrative of cultural exoneration and continue to haunt us, their wounds, and ours, shall remain raw.

BIBLIOGRAPHY

Barthes, Roland. 1973. *Le Plaisir du texte*. Paris: Seuil.

Boulé, Jean-Pierre. 2002. *HIV Stories: The Archeology of AIDS Writing in France: 1985–1988*. Liverpool: University of Liverpool Press.

BPM [*120 battements par minute*]. 2017. Dir. Robin Campillo. Memento Films. Film.

Chambers, Ross. 1998. *Facing I: AIDS Diaries and the Death of the Author*. Ann Arbor: The University of Michigan Press.

———. 2004. *Untimely Interventions: AIDS Writing, Testimonial, and the Rhetoric of Haunting*. Ann Arbor, The University of Michigan Press.

Daney, Serge. 1996. *La rampe: Cahier critique 1970–1982*. Paris: Gallimard.

———. 1997. *Devant la recrudescence des vols de sacs à main*. Paris: Aléas.

Dean, Tim. 2009. *Unlimited Intimacy: Reflections on the Subculture of Barebacking*. Chicago: University of Chicago Press.

Dustan, Guillaume. 1996. *In My Room*. Trans. Brad Rumph. London: Serpent's Tail, 1998. Trans. Of *Dans ma chambre*. Paris: P.O.L.

Genton, Camille. 2017. *Positif*. Paris: JC Lattès.

Guibert, Hervé. 1990. *To the Friend Who Did Not Save My Life*. Trans. Linda Coverdale. New York: Atheneum, 1991. Trans. of *A l'ami qui ne m'a pas sauvé la vie*. Paris: Gallimard.

———. 1992. *Cytomegalovirus: A Hospitalization Diary*. Trans. Clara Orban. New York: Fordham University Press, 2016. Trans. of *Cytomégalovirus: Journal d'hospitalisation*. Paris: Seuil.

Hovhannessian, Lucie. 2018. *Presque comme les autres: ma vie de jeune séropositive*. Paris: Robert Laffont.

How to Survive a Plague. 2012. Dir. David France. GathrFilms, Film.

Lévi-Strauss, Claude. 1964. *Le cru et le cuit*. Paris: Plon.

Marquart, Sharon. 2015. *On the Defensive: Reading the Ethical in Nazi Camp Testimonies*. Toronto: University of Toronto Press.

Race, Kane. 2010. "Engaging in a Culture of Barebacking: Gay Men and the Risk of HIV Prevention." *HIV Treatment and Prevention Technologies in International Perspective*. Ed. by Mark Davis and Corinne Squire. London: Palgrave Macmillan, 144–66.

Simonin, Michel. 1986. *Danger de vie*. Paris: Librairie Séguier.

Tomso, Gregory. 2008. "Viral Sex and the Politics of Life. *South Atlantic Quarterly* 107:2: 265–85.

Trezise, Thomas. 2013. *Witnessing Witnessing: On the Reception of Holocaust Survivor Testimony*. New York: Fordham University Press.

United in Anger: A History of ACT UP. 2012. Dir. Jim Hubbard. No distributor. Film.

NOTES

1. Predictably, HIV writing has mirrored the demographic shifts of the epidemic. In the United States, for example, where HIV incidence has remained an intractable problem in some African-American communities, black voices have made themselves heard in ways that weren't always possible when white gay men and homophobes were fighting for discursive supremacy in the public arena.

2. "[F]ace à la crudité-naturalisme (Renoir), à la crudité-impressionnisme (Bresson) ou à la crudité-art moderne (Godard), on retrouve toujours le mijoté à la Tavernier ou le frichti Berri" (*Devant la recrudescence des vols de sacs à main*, 96). ["Facing rawness-as-naturalism (Renoir), rawness-as-impressionism (Bresson) and rawness-as-modern-art (Godard), you'll always find a Tavernier stew or a Berri chow."]

3. Community also permeates Guibert's and Dustan's seminal books on AIDS. *A l'ami* depicts what we could call an AIDS community comprising all sorts of people whose lives have been upended by the crisis, while *Dans ma chambre* focuses on the gay community, both local and global, affected by AIDS.

4. The Treatment Action Group, or TAG, was formed in 1992, when members of ACT UP-New York's Treatment and Data Committee decided to start their own organization focused on research for HIV treatments.

5. Access to bank loans is no trivial matter, as the long history of denying them to African-Americans keeps reminding us.

6. In 2018, Camille Genton appeared in a video for Emmanuel Macron's party En marche for a "Journée contre le sida."

7. I thank Steven Kurtz for this insight.

8. The movie streams on Kanopy.

Chapter Two

Raw Writing

AIDS Autofiction and the Construction of Seropositive Subjectivity

V. Hunter Capps

THE GENRE OF THE RAW

I seek here to explore what I will call raw writing. It will come to represent a genre and style of writing deployed by seropositive individuals that utilized queer excess in the form of sex, the body, language, and drugs in order to both make intelligible new subjectivities brought about by HIV/AIDS as well as to manifest or perform the very potentiality inherent to literature and the act of writing. First and foremost, this endeavor requires an intake of definitions. Deriving from the Old English, *hreaw* was used to speak of food. The leading definition of the word simply means "not cooked" (Merriam Webster). Concerning the French "cru," the other etymological root from the Latin *crudus* is also of importance as it gestures toward that which is "marked by absence of refinements" (Ibid.). The word is also cited as meaning, "in a natural state; not yet processed or worked" (Ibid.). More than just food or fabric, however, raw is used similarly when discussing emotions wherein a transitional movement is invoked as raw emotions become filtered through rationality or reason. Raw is also somewhat synonymously associated with a sense of risk. Many restaurants that serve a variety of cuisines whose components are best served with minimal acts of cooking are usually required by law to state somewhere on their menus that the consumption of undercooked or raw foods could potentially expose one to food-borne illnesses.

Nevertheless, this risk, much like we will see later in the context of sex, rarely stops people from the appeal of enjoying a rare steak, sushi, or an over-easy egg. Indeed, overcooking or over-processing certain foods or fabrics comes with its own variety of pitfalls that can leave a palate, culinary or otherwise, wanting more. Another definition of the word is, “not being in polished, finished, or processed form” (Ibid.), as is the case with raw data. Yet another definition is, “having the surface abraded or chafed; very irritated” (Ibid.), such as rubbing one’s skin raw. Implicit in these understandings of raw is a separation of time, space, and substance all of which quite sensitively inform an overall idea of rawness. Something exists in a natural or primitive state and is thus described as raw only after a sense of movement and action is invoked. Definitions of when and where raw is exactly demarcated are then subject to varying mechanisms that are used to process or filter the object at hand. Raw then is wrapped up both in its descriptive capacities as well as its fluctuating methods that describe these states of being. In other words, rawness can be understood as both in matters of content as well as in matters of method(ology), and both are intimately bound up with each other. In short, where and when the boundaries of rawness are constituted is dependent on the substance at hand (flesh, food, fabric) as well as its relative temporal relationship (before/after) to the mechanisms (tearing, cooking, dying) that could possibly be applied. With these definitions in mind, I wish to examine the use of autofiction as a queer genre-bending kind of writing utilized by HIV-positive writers who took up autofiction as a means to explore their seropositivity as well as the social and biomedical ravages of HIV. My goal is to demonstrate how such writing and those behind it helped to elaborate on and spread new forms of queer knowledge that have reshaped the parameters of sex, desire, and communities.

Apropos of the question of genre, the tension between memoir and (auto) fiction speaks to how the latter seemingly understands the impossibility of succinct memory, choosing instead to embrace and exploit fissures and gaps to imagine a present/past that is not as debilitating as its “real” counterpart. Otherwise stated, autofiction queerly and thus performatively participates in a fantasy that imagines elsewhere/wise, blurring the time of the writing, the time of the text, and the time of the reading which ultimately is what animates it and gives it life. Jason Tougaw notes:

> It [this new subject of writing] threatens, through the violation of conventional boundaries between Self and Other (both literally, through bodily exchange, and figuratively, through total psychic identification), to *infect* the culture at large; it charts new social relations, in which AIDS is no longer incomprehensible but a full-fledged social problem, with a language and structure that can “accommodate” people with AIDS. (2002, 175, original emphasis)

Monica Pearl similarly observes that, "The hybrid nature of the texts, the fact that they rely on different genres to produce the whole, mark the texts as impure, or infected" (2012, 72). For Tougaw, his emphasis is on the subject of the genre while Pearl's is on genre itself. In these formulations, both authors rely on a rather salient metaphor of infection to classify AIDS writing and its subjects. The reader inevitably becomes infected by way of the performative gesture of reading the text, but the reader is not so much infected with literal HIV as he is with the knowledge that accompanies introspection of the disease and the irreversible trauma it wrought. Indeed, as Tougaw highlights, "The virus travels between us because our bodies (like our psyches) are permeable, and the bodily infection spreads, signifying both corporeal and psychic connections between us" (2002, 172). Thus, if we maintain the logic underlying risk assessment with respect to raw gay sex, and we understand that reading these texts runs the risk of infecting us with HIV knowledge, then such a model of risk holds up when applied to literature, for seeking out knowledge is indeed always going to be a risky endeavor that, like sex, can also produce pleasure.

(T)-MINUS . . .

Hervé Guibert most notably came into the public eye with the publication of his novel *À l'ami qui ne m'a pas sauvé la vie* (1990) [*To the Friend Who Did Not Save My Life* (1991)] in which he utilized autofiction to recount living with AIDS. Indeed, from the start of the novel, there is no mistake that AIDS is at the center of the story. Dryly, rawly, and declaratively stated, the first words of the first chapter are, "J'ai eu le sida pendant trois mois" (9) [I had AIDS for three months (1)]. Well-educated and culturally associated with the likes of Roland Barthes, Isabelle Adjani, and Michel Foucault, Guibert took himself seriously as a writer and took up writing as a sort of treatment for himself. In *Le protocole compassionnel* (1991) [*The Compassion Protocol* (1993)], his second popular text that treated his suffering from AIDS, he says, "C'est quand j'écris que je suis le plus vivant" (124) [It's when I'm writing that I feel most alive (106)]. When it comes to Guibert, and later as I will show with Guillaume Dustan, we see a gay, HIV-positive subject attempting to remember, recount, or simply just account for his suffering from a disease that has been directly associated with his sexual identity. In turning to autofiction, such a literary endeavor can be seen as the creating of oneself a fiction from raw materials. It is always an exploration wherein the "I" of the author and the "I" of the narrator become tenuous, a place where literature allows for safe haven and introspection. Indeed, for Guibert, it becomes a life-affirming task, a necessary labor that keeps his frail and dying existence alive. More to the point, Guibert uses autofiction as a site wherein he even derives a certain pleasure by reflecting on his suffering and HIV-infected existence.

Throughout the text of *The Compassion Protocol*, Guibert constantly references a certain supply of a drug called DDI (Didanosine) that he came into possession of through the black market because the previous owner, a dancer, had succumbed to HIV. Guibert is bound to the hopefully life-saving drug by way of the dancer's haunting presence that is inextricably associated with the drug. I want to focus on a specific excerpt wherein Guibert references the DDI in meticulous detail while also relating the drug's positive effects with his ability and drive to write. He writes: C'est le DDI du danseur mort, avec le Prozac, qui écrit mon livre, à ma place. Ce sont ces 335 milligrammes de poudre blanche fabriqué à Ickenham, Middlesex, en Angleterre, et cette gélule quotidienne de 20 milligrammes de Fluoxétine Chlorhydrate qui me redonnent la force de vivre, d'espérer; de bander, de bander pour la vie, et d'écrire (1991, 84) [It's the dead ballet dancer's DDI, with Prozac, writing my book for me. It is these 335 milligrams of white powder manufactured in England at Ickenham, Middlesex, and this daily capsule of 20 milligrams of Fluoxetine Chlorhydrate that are giving back the strength to stay alive, to hope; to get a hard on, to get hard for dear life, and to write (1993, 69)]. The drug and its effects are cited not solely as inspiration for Guibert's writing but rather as the authors themselves. There is a certain intimacy with which Guibert describes in precise detail the dosages, quality, and origin of his drugs. More interesting still, the particular amounts of these specific drugs are also said to be that which has revitalized Guibert not simply just to live but to be sexually aroused. While the medications have brought about a new, hopeful outlook on life, they have also reawakened Guibert's sexual drive. Guibert directly associates this sexual arousal then with being aroused for life, and from here is where he ends up at the ultimate verb in his sequence: "écrire" [to write]. Writing, understood in this specific context as autofiction as a means to account, to bear witness to one's own suffering, also becomes a site of life-giving and life-affirming pleasure. In the same sentence where we see death and suffering, we also see life born anew with sexual vivacity. For a gay man dying of a political disease associated with his sexual practices, this new take on life must indeed be sexual.

Dagmawi Woubshet notes how in AIDS writing "a trope of inventory taking surfaces time and again as a haunting leifmotif" (2015, 3). Pearl also elaborates on this leitmotif by stating that "Everything is articulated, nothing held back. There are no detectable elisions of story or identity. With such imminent losses there is a tendency to believe . . . that if everything is articulated the losses might be stemmed, or sufficiently memorialized" (2012, 28). With respect to my argument about raw writing, it is thus worthy of note that this context of inventory taking represents raw data ("335 milligrams,"

"20 milligrams") used to document Guibert's life-saving drugs, a vital role in his continued survival. Elsewhere, this raw materiality is well documented in Guibert's writing as he obsessively tracks his T-cell count while it slowly keeps dropping. It is a symbol for the slow progression of the virus that becomes a way for the reader to more directly associate with the existential suffering of the narrator/author. We see the first documentation of Guibert's T-cells early on in *To the Friend* where he says: "Les dernières analyses, datées du 18 novembre, me donnent 368 T4" (1990, 13) [My most recent test results, dated November 18, show a T4 count of 368] (1991, 5). Later, it seems as if things are looking up when he says: "je me trouvais en fait dans un phase de répit et même de repli de cette maladie car mon niveau de T4 était remonté à plus de 550" (2017) [at the moment when I'd felt so weakened by my illness, the disease had actually been in remission, because my T4 count had risen to more than 550] (176). Toward the end of the text, however, Guibert finds himself arriving at the crucial T-cell threshold for which he could be considered in the vaccine trials that Bill, the eponymous friend had promised: "car le 12 janvier le docteur Chandi m'a révélé au téléphone que leur taux avait chuté à 291, en un mois de 368 à 291, ce qui peut laisser penser qu'après un mois supplementaire d'offensive du virus HIV [sic] à l'intérieur de mon sang mon taux de T4 n'en est plus qu'à (je fais la soustraction au bas de cette page) 213" (232) [because on January 12 Dr. Chandi told me over the phone that my T4 count had dropped to 291, from 368 to 291 in one month, which suggests that in another month, the HIV virus [sic] will have ground my T4 count down to—I'm doing the subtraction at the bottom of the page—214 [sic]] (197–8). And later still, "Les candidats ne doivent avoir subi aucun traitement, et avoir plus de 200 T4. Les toutes dernières analyses m'en donnent 200 pile" (269) [The candidates must not have undergone any treatment, and must have a T4 count above 200. My latest lab report gives me 200 on the nose] (233).

What is significant to understand in these passages wherein Guibert tracks his T-cell count is what is suggested in such documentation. What Guibert refers to as T4s are a group of T-cells subdivided into what in common HIV parlance are known as CD4s. These are the white blood cells that HIV attacks and depletes which in turn lowers the bodily defenses that fend off infection. When an HIV-positive person descends to 200 CD4s per cubic millimeter of blood is when that person is technically diagnosed as having AIDS ("AIDS Case Definition" 2019). Guibert himself refers to it as "le seuil fatal" (1990, 195) [the fatal threshold] (1991, 167). If we are to understand the depletion of CD4s not simply as an advancement of the virus but also as a continuous erosion of the bodily defenses and thus a greater vulnerability, we could also say that we see Guibert become more and more raw to us the readers. Or, at the very least, his suffering is put on raw display, and it is through his writing about it that we too pass this critical threshold. However, for us it is not the amount of CD4s in our blood but instead the extent of our exposure to Guibert's suffering and his subjectivity. Remember that for Guibert, writing is indissociable from his will to live which in turn is intimately bound up with his sexual drive and desire. It is thus that we must understand that our exposure to his writing, our exposure to his feeble blood and body is always already wrapped up in a complicated circuit wherein sex, pleasure, desire, death, and suffering are intimately intertwined.

In *AIDS in French Culture,* David Caron develops an idea of "diseased discourse" that emerges out of AIDS writing and its subjects. It draws parallels between the fractured subject of Guibert's suffering in autofiction and the fractured subject position that any postmodern subject can inhabit in discourse. Indeed, the discourse, the raw material of this diseased subject's constitution, impregnated with this new seropositive perspective becomes metaphorically as infectious as the disease that brought about its existence. Caron writes that "By equating reading and fucking, Guibert reminds his readers that we too may be engaging in risky behavior . . . the reader may in turn become contaminated by reading Guibert" (2001, 139). Guibert makes his suffering palpable by inevitably exposing us, through his raw writing, to his seropositive subjectivity from which we cannot return uncontaminated. Not only are we as readers learning about the raw material that constitutes the parameters of this illness and its effects on the body, but we are also intimately exposed to the perspective of the one who is under assault as he must slowly write his way toward his inevitable death.

In *The Compassion Protocol*, after resolving himself to no longer caring where his T-cell count rests, "Je ne veux plus savoir où j'en suis, je ne le demande plus au médecin, ni à voir les résultats des analyses qu'on a pris l'habitude, avec le sida" (1991, 167) [I no longer want to know what point I have reached, I no longer ask the doctor what my level is, no longer want to see the results of the tests that you get so used to having done when you have 'the Big A' [sic]] (1993, 143), Guibert works himself back around to understanding how the constant confrontation with his mortality has forever shifted his perspective: "Je suis dans une zone de menace où je voudrais plutôt me donner l'illusion de la survie, et de la vie éternelle. Oui, il me faut bien l'avouer et je crois que c'est le sort commun de tous les grands malades, même si c'est pitoyable et ridicule, après avoir tant rêvé à la mort, dorénavant j'ai horriblement envie de vivre." (167) [I'm in a constantly threatened zone in which I would rather allow myself the illusion of survival, of eternal life. Yes, I have to admit it and I think it's the common destiny of all the seriously ill, even if it sounds pitiable and ridiculous, after dreaming so much of dying, from now on I only have a horrible yearning to go on living] (143). Fully admitting to himself and the reader the "pitiful" and "ridiculous" nature of his stance, the narrator/author dismisses such absurdity in the face of his raw desire to simply live. With respect to how the definition of raw is temporally marked and subject to a transition from one state to another, the usage of "dorénavant [from now on]" is important as it reinforces the temporal aspect of Guibert's sentiments and thus the rawness of his desire. There is a before when all Guibert could do was dream about death, track his falling T-cells, watch his body waste away, but now the desperation, dread, and rawness hang from the adverb "horriblement [horrible]" as Guibert insists that he simply wants to continue living. As was the case with so many of the queer ancestors like him, Guibert did not get his wish and died on December 27, 1991, a substantial distance of five years before life-saving medication became available.

RAW IS LAW: THE DUSTANIEN TEXT

In 1996, fifteen years into the epidemic, scientific institutions were able to test, reproduce, and market antiretroviral medication, more colloquially known as tri-therapy, that successfully prevented HIV from replicating. Viral loads went down, CD4s went up, and some people most literally came back from the brink of death. As people began to recuperate not only from the disease but also from the social weight of losing friends and family, the conversations about HIV and sex began to shift. HIV was most certainly not curable, but for those living in a Western country like France whose healthcare system guaranteed treatment, HIV no longer carried the burden of death with it that plagued Guibert and those like him who did not make it to 1996. More interestingly still, what to make of those who willingly abandoned condoms and participated in raw sex in the face of tri-therapy? A shift in consciousness concerning seropositivity and queerness began to take place in 1996, and for a writer like Guillaume Dustan, he was tackling what seemed like an almost entirely new problem when it came to sex, desire, and the experiences formed around them, especially with respect to a minoritarian community of people that had seen firsthand the ravages of HIV. Infected in 1990, Dustan was no stranger to the height of the plague days that saw his friends, lovers, and his neighborhood pillaged by the disease and political indifference. In *Dans ma chambre* ([1996] 2013) [*In My Room* (1998)], Dustan says, "Ça fait quatre ans déjà que je pense que je vais mourir l'année prochaine. Je me trouve beau quand même" (62) [It's been four years now that I've been thinking I am to die the next year. I think I still look handsome though] (1998, 25). More to the point, Dustan, like Guibert, was subject to facing his mortality in ways that harbored no promise, for he could not have seen the dawn of tri-therapy in 1996 to come. Nevertheless, Dustan utilized his experiences as a seropositive gay man who actively desired not just sex but raw gay sex as a main vehicle to tell his stories and explore the new terrain of queer excess, queer desire, and queer kinship that came with living in a post-AIDS Parisian world. For my purposes here, I employ "post-AIDS" to specifically denote a time after tri-therapy so as to speak on the complex sociopolitical matters that arose once AIDS, an outdated term whose meaning carries with it the lingering ignorance originally born around the disease, became treatable to the extent that people could survive simply as HIV-positive.[1] "AIDS" then comes to signify a specific time that begins in 1981 when the disease is acknowledged, through the tumultuous sixteen years when no effective treatment existed and people were dying en masse, and "ends" in 1996 with the arrival of tri-therapy. HIV, of course, did not end, but a new chapter in thought concerning the disease began.

Before directly delving into the content of Dustan's writing, it is worthwhile to contextualize the atmosphere in which his novels emerged as well as the reactions to the novels so that when addressing his work I am able to more clearly show how crucial his writing was in the advancement of queer thought. In 1989, Act Up-Paris was formed and much like its American counterpart (ACT UP) spent its political endeavors fighting the government for lack of action at the level of prevention. Known for their aggressive political tactics, ACT UP was irrefutably crucial in the fight against AIDS both in America and France. For the French manifestation of ACT UP, prevention was always at the forefront of their concerns. The socialist French government under the rule of François Mitterrand had minimized statutes criminalizing homosexuality, yet they failed to act in a way that properly addressed the epidemic. There were several contributing factors, but the largest was France's universalist stance on citizenship that saw the erasure and rejection of communitarian-based politics.[2] Noble as the efforts of Act Up-Paris were, with tri-therapy available, Act Up-Paris began to lose steam and their political effectiveness began to wane. The group even coined the term *le relapse* to discuss issues surrounding the willful abandonment of condoms, and I think it is of particular rhetorical importance to examine the function that such a word plays in a conversation concerning HIV. Relapse, an English word appropriated into a French context, implies a certain falling back into a behavior, usually that of drug use, a social ill not seen as anything more than an unfortunate vice. With respect to the temporal definition of raw I have been maintaining, this temporally sensitive word used to discuss raw gay sex is particularly interesting as relapse seems also to suggest a moment of respite wherein condoms were welcomed, embraced, and condomless sex stopped. While condom usage of course went up during the crisis given the prominence of "safe sex" discourse, the number of seroconversions themselves speaks to the fact that condoms were not necessarily embraced with enthusiasm. Moreover, the usage of "relapse" seems to suggest an inherent flaw in those who did choose to abandon condoms. Indeed, I think it is of paramount importance to relate the usage of the term to the emergence of effective treatment since in the eyes of Act Up-Paris it was such treatment that apparently allowed for the falling back into condomless behavior. What Act Up-Paris seemed to miss was that to condemn condomless sex was itself a futile, demonizing gesture that in the end did not achieve the political outcomes it was seeking but rather took a moralizing high ground that further pointed the finger at gay men for being responsible not only for their own seroconversions but for the epidemic writ large.

"Baiser sans capote ça vous fait jouir?" [Does Condomless Sex Make You Come?] was the slogan used in an Act Up-Paris campaign in 1999 specifically targeted at the growing popularity at the time of "barebackers" as well as Erik Rémès who also openly discussed condomless sex. Guillaume Dustan had garnered the ire of Act Up-Paris over the years but more specifically because he, in the eyes of Act Up-Paris, dared to speak about sex without the latex prophylactic that was considered to be the only barrier between the community and the death that had plagued them from 1981 to 1996. Perhaps not so ironically, Act Up-Paris's slogan points not just to the fallacy of their intentions with the campaign, arguably nothing short of scare tactics, but perhaps more pointedly to the rhetorical answer to the proposed question. Indeed, fucking without condoms does make one come, as they admit in the small blurb at the bottom of the posters, which begs the question as to what the group truly meant by such a rhetorical formulation. I might argue that the response Act Up-Paris wanted to illicit from this slogan was that sex without condoms *should not* make one aroused, and to take it a step further, one should prevent oneself from even desiring such a thing because despite successful drug treatments, there still existed the *risk* of contamination. It is as if gay men were forever barred, because of pure risk alone, from ever experiencing the pleasure and intimacy that comes with raw sex, and to even desire such a thing was strictly forbidden. The aggressiveness in this rhetorical posturing reflects Act Up-Paris's historically combative attitude that propelled them into the spotlight of international news as well as communitarian leadership. However, the slogan is also emblematic of the one-track mindedness of the organization that spent years trying to obtain dignified treatment for those living with HIV once such medication had become available.[3]

Toward the end of the poster's paragraph, they write "Pour notre part, nous n'arrivons pas à mettre à côté notre expérience du sida. Nous n'arrivons pas à jouir sans capote. Le risque de contaminer ou d'être contaminé continue de gâcher notre plaisir" (1999) ["For us, we are unable to put aside our experience of AIDS. We are unable to cum without condoms. The risk of contaminating or of being contaminated continues to spoil our pleasure"] (my translation). It is worthwhile to stop and interrogate exactly who this first-person plural "we" is that Act Up-Paris is invoking here. It would appear that they are speaking for the organization first but perhaps even the gay community as a whole. The reactionary tone creates a divide in the community between those who can apparently put AIDS behind them, whatever that might mean, and those who cannot: the mindless, amoral barebackers versus the noble, scarred soldiers of the plague days. This false dichotomy is all too emblematic of Act Up-Paris' misgivings that led them so deep into a radical politic so as to deface the literature of whom they saw as their opponents.[4] But what was so scary about raw sex that would propel Act Up-Paris into such totalitarian territory? What did these authors do or say that put the group so on the defensive against their own people? Drawing heavily on Guillaume Dustan, I would like to argue that his extension of the genre of autofiction in the form of raw writing challenged not only the safe sex rhetoric of Act Up-Paris and the State, but it also pushed the boundaries of sex, desire, and risk beyond simple definitions of permissible sexual acts and behavior. Dustan utilized autofiction as a means to explore the shifting landscape of queer emotion and desire in the face of a politically imbued viral genocide that slowly but surely deteriorated the body and the mind and eventually a large portion of a minority community. Sometimes palpably present and other times only haunting the text, rawness, or raw gay sex, plays a role in how the raw writers were able to navigate their desires and themselves.

"GAYTTO" LIVING

As stated in the recently published biography on his life, "Son vrai nom est William Baranès. Il est juif, pédé, séropo (dans l'ordre d'apparition de ces phénomènes dans sa vie). Magistrat, juriste à l'occasion, écrivain, éditeur et même vidéaste" (Enault 2018, 14–5) ["His real name is William Baranès. He is a Jew, a fag, and poz (in order of these phenomena's appearances in his life). Magistrate, legal expert, writer, editor, and even video maker"] (my translation). Baranès did not become Dustan until 1994 when he began his experimental foray into literature. Heralded as an intellectual prodigy in his youth, Baranès eventually pursued his studies to the level of becoming an énarque (a graduate of the prestigious École Nationale de l'Administration [National School of Administration]). Unlike Guibert who took himself to be a serious writer, Dustan came to writing to utilize it as an experimental force irrespective of French literary conventions.[5] In *Dans ma chambre*, Dustan picks up the genre of autofiction and takes the reader on a whirlwind ride through a plethora of sex, drugs, and partying. His second text, *Je sors ce soir* ([1997] 2013) [*I'm Going Out Tonight*][6] sees the author/narrator traverse one wild night of Parisian nightlife. The prose of the books is simple, direct, and uncomplicated with short sentences, lucid language, and a simple overlying structure. The title of the first novel itself signals a problematic of the public/private divide that the AIDS crisis, especially in France, seriously troubled. We as the readers are invited into the intimate space of Dustan's room/life where his sexual escapades and excessive behavior are put on full display.

The backdrop of his stories is Le Marais, the gay *and* Jewish district of Paris that, because of its homogenized minority communities, is often referred to as the ghetto or even "gaytto." Before continuing with any analysis of Dustan's texts, this language needs to be unpacked in order to fully understand the historical, cultural, and linguistic weight of the term. There has been much debate about the use of the word "ghetto," but for my purposes I draw on the Italian root meaning "foundry," an original location where Jews' living space was restricted (Merriam-Webster).[7] This root is of course what informed the more contemporary understanding of the word that derives from the Nazi practices of racializing Jews during World War II. Given the French collaboration with the Nazis during the war and the vehement retaliation against those collaborators after liberation, the term has a particular resonance in French contexts. Keeping in mind the role of French Republicanism in the AIDS crisis, that governing modus operandi that sees over-identifying with communitarian identity as leading to ghettoization and thus a fracturing of national unity, the appropriation of the term "ghetto" by a HIV-positive, French, gay Jew to take pride in his decidedly contrarian and queer identity is incredibly layered and signals that the impetus for such an appropriation has to do with more than just the literal boundaries of the Marais. It is also worthy to note, with respect to parallels between the utterances of the word, that the French gay community that was localized in the Marais did indeed see mass death of its community members as well. Moreover, Dustan's embrasure and appropriation of the word is one thing, but its usage extends beyond a simple conversation about a literal place/space. Oliver Davis notes that "the bareback writer would characterize members of Act Up and others who also believed in imposing their norm of compulsory condom use more emotively still as 'kapos of the ghetto'" (2015, 150). Once more, a historical line is drawn upon to conceptually frame the debate around Act Up-Paris and the bareback authors. By framing the actions of Didier Lestrade and his colleagues as being akin to those working in Nazi concentration camps, an emphasis is put on the inter-community role that Act Up-Paris had in policing the actions of its own members.

Located in the city center right off the Seine, the Marais provides a particularly French as well as a particularly queer setting for the events in Dustan's novels wherein we see a profound sense of queer kinship develop that is heavily rooted in space and the bodies that come into contact there. In *Dans ma chambre*, in a chapter entitled, in English, "People are still having sex,"

Dustan proudly declares his admiration of the ghetto: "Je vis dans un monde merveilleux où tout le monde a couhcé avec tout le monde . . . On a le choix. Beaucoup de choix. Et personne ne souhaite fonder une famille. On est un, ou deux, pas plus, dans ce monde, sauf quand il y a pour un temps plus ou moins long un esclave à la maison. Je trouve ça bien toute cette invention" ([1996] 2013, 81) ["I live in a wonderful world where the whole world has been to bed with the whole world . . . take your pick. You've got a lot to pick from. And nobody's looking to start a family. You are one or no more than two in this world except when there's a slave at home for a more or less long time. I think it's fine all this inventiveness"] (1998, 52). This marvelous world of Dustan, a reflection of its real counterpart, is populated by an expansive and diverse group of men who have all seemingly slept with each other, and such connections are what form the bond of a specific kind of queer kinship. He declaratively states the radically queer nature of this community's desires and interests but not without a crass and humorous tone as he gestures to the idea of keeping around sexual slaves. Later still, he writes: "On est bien dans le ghetto. Il y a du monde . . . À part bosser, en général, et voir sa famille, tout peut se faire sans sortir du ghetto" (83) ["We're doing fine in the ghetto. There's a lot of people . . . Apart from the job, in general, and seeing the family, everything can be done without going out of the ghetto"] (55–6). The outskirts of the Marais, the land of the heteros, is dangerous and undesirable whereas the confines of the ghetto provide safety and intimate bonds of pleasure and kinship, a reappropriated inverse of the original meaning of the word.

This kinship, heavily defined through sex, is not however without its implications of AIDS and death. In a chapter entitled, in English again, "Living in the ghetto," Dustan recounts a scene in a club that begins with a conversation about dead friends: "Dimanche soir à Loco je suis tombé sur Tom. Il m'a dit que son ex était mort" (79) ["Sunday night at the Loco I ran into Tom. He told me his ex was dead"] (50). Death is foregrounded and hovers over the interactions between the men in the bar. A few lines later we read, "Pendant le dîner Stéphane a appris qu'un type qu'il connaissait de l'Asmf est mort" (79) ["At dinner Stéphane found out a guy he knew from Act-up [sic] is dead"] (50). Dustan is not unaware of this weight that hangs over the community. Later in the chapter he says, "J'étais déjà déprimé" (79) ["I was already depressed"] (50) before he loses his temper with Stéphane and lets out his sexual frustrations: "excuses-moi en ce moment je suis déprimé, je préférais que tu me baises. Ou alors je te baise sans capote. Il m'a dit Baise-moi sans capote. J'ai rebandé instantanément . . . au bout de cinq minutes évidemment j'avais envie de jouir alors que d'habitude avec une capote ça ne vient jamais tellement je reste à distance" (79) ["excuse me but right now I'm depressed, I'd rather you fuck me. Or else I'd fuck you without a condom. He said Fuck me without a condom. Instantly my hard-on sprang back . . . Five minutes later of course I was ready to cum, whereas, with a condom on I usually never do, I'm at such a distance"] (51). Although sex is celebrated if not glorified in this community, it is accompanied by the constant specter of death. We see how Dustan's depression turns into immediate sexual excitation once the prospect of raw sex is proposed while he ruminates on the immense difference between sex with and without a condom. In no way do we see him promoting condomless sex, but rather we see an honest, raw take on the nature of desire with respect to gay sex in a world saturated with AIDS-related death.

With each new chapter, we see Dustan engaged in some sort of new sexual escapade either with his temporary partner Stéphane or some other person he has come across online or in the clubs. The descriptions of these scenes, mostly with condoms though not all, are emblematic of the raw quality of Dustan's writing because his gory details actually reflect the reality of gay life. For example, Dustan does not shy away from the more unseemly side of anal sex among men. He often speaks about douching, the act of cleaning out one's colon, a detail far removed from other romantic, arguably more heteronormative, depictions of gay love elsewhere. In a chapter simply titled "Sex," once more in English, a scene unfolds where after having done cocaine and smoking hash, Dustan sends Stéphane to the bathroom before they get down to business: "Je l'envoie chier et se laver le cul" (57) ["I send him off to shit and wash his ass"] (18). Later, in a scene that I want to cite at length so as to get a sense of his uninterrupted, rapid-fire prose, we see how the method of his writing brings to life the intensity, the rawness of his content:

> je me lève et je vais me laver le cul dans la sale de bains, je donne pas d'explications puisqu'il entend les bruits, ça me prend un bon moment, quand je reviens je suis un peu désexcité alors je refais un pétard, on le fume en regardant la télé et puis je redescends sur la bite de Stéphane et quand il est bien dur je me mets sur le dos et j'écarte les jambes et il vient sur moi et il me saute en profondeur avec une compréhension parfaite de mes entrailles, je bande comme un fou sans me toucher, vingt minutes je pense, je le caresse, je lui fais les seins, je presse ma bite gonflée contre son ventre, il me fait un truc que j'adore faire aussi, il roule son ventre contre mes couilles en me baisant. Multiplication de points sensibles. (59)
>
> [I get up and go wash out my ass in the bathroom. I give no explanation for the noises he can hear. It takes me a while, and when I come back I'm not turned on as much so I roll another joint, we smoke it watching TV and then I go back down on his dick and when he's real hard I get on my back and I spread my legs and he gets on top and pokes me deep, with a perfect comprehension of my entrails, my dick is rock hard without my touching, twenty minutes I think, I fondle him, I squeeze his tits, I press my expanding dick up against his abs,

> he does a trick I love doing too, he roles his abs against my balls fucking me. Multiplication of the sensitive points.] (21–2)

This paragraph-long sentence, describing how the sex takes place, functions to demonstrate the raw quality of the content since we are spared no detail of the acts taking place. Moreover, the form of its delivery renders the material all the rawer. In the original French, commas separate a constant stream of independent clauses, actions, and thoughts while at times they are all rammed together, much like Dustan in the scene himself, separated only by a series of and's. The scene leaves the reader breathless both from the content covered as well as the way it was delivered as if we the readers were also fucked as intensely as Dustan was.

Toward the end of his second book *Je sors ce soir,* after having had a few drinks, smoked a few spliffs, and taken a dose of ecstasy, Dustan utilizes the structure of the text and space of the page in a manner common to poetry but not as often used in prose. As the drugs begin to kick in, his sentences become short and separated by line. He acknowledges that with the onset of the drugs, he is not thinking of dead friends, past lovers, possibly infecting an old partner; he is escaping this crippling reality. We then see the raw form of the writing begin to express his raw state of mind. The next page is comprised of three hyper short sentences, the next only two, and the following only one. Then nothing. Fourteen blank pages follow that presumably represent Dustan having lost consciousness for an indiscernible amount of time ([1997] 2013, 200–14). In the empty space of these blank pages we see the respite the excessive drug use has brought Dustan as we the readers are also forced to confront what such silence entails. More interestingly still, by the fourteenth blank page we can see the text to come through the page itself, however that text on the other side is blurred and amorphous. It is nevertheless visible, thus signaling a return to consciousness on the horizon. As we turn the page and can then make out the text, we, like Dustan, are thrust headfirst back into reality. This method of utilizing the literal space of the page to enhance the experience of the content which is itself rooted in the excess of drug use in a gay space stands out as a truly remarkable facet of Dustan's writing and exemplary of the raw capacities of literature.

Guibert slowly tracked his T-cell depletion and thus his death to the point that it gave him a new lease on life. Dustan's narcotic and sexual excesses allowed for a brief impression of a marvelous and fulfilling world before his own mortality caught up with him. In each case, we are offered a raw glimpse into the shifting landscape of queer identity and desire in the wake of HIV, a new harbinger of death now inextricably bound to gay ontology and queer politics. By harnessing the imaginative space of literature, both seropositive gay men offered up their subjectivities as a means through which we readers might be able to understand the new parameters of queer life. Death, now wrapped up in HIV and sexual politics, provided the groundwork upon which queers yet again managed to build life anew. Furthermore, by not tailoring them to be palatable to a heteronormative sensibility, by presenting these experiences raw as they came, and by utilizing the raw capacities of writing these authors were able to simultaneously bear witness to a generation of gay men left to die as well as lend cultural intelligibility to a subjectivity that would forever alter the landscape of queerness.

BIBLIOGRAPHY

Agar, James N. 2011. "Queer in France: AIDS Disidentification in France." In *Queer in Europe: Contemporary Case Studies*, edited by Robert Gillett and Lisa Downing, 57–70. London: Routledge.

"AIDS Case Definition." National Institutes of Health U.S. Department of Health and Human Services, accessed November 2019, http://aidsinfo.nih.gov/understanding-hiv-aids/glossary/2925/aids-case-definition.

"Baiser sans capote ça vous fait jouir?" 1999. AIDS Education Collection; Department of Rare Books, Special Collections, and Preservation; River Campus Libraries, University of Rochester.

Bosia, Michal J. 2006. "'Assassin!' AIDS and Neoliberal Reform in France." *New Political Science* 27, No. 3 (August): 291–308.

Boulé, Jean-Pierre. 2002. *HIV Stories: The Archaeology of AIDS Writing in France.* Liverpool: Liverpool University Press.

Broqua, Christophe. [2005] 2020. *Action=Vie: A History of AIDS Activism and Gay Politics in France*. Trans. by Jean-Yves Bart and Kel Pero. Philadelphia: Temple University Press.

Butler, Paul. 2004. "Embracing AIDS: History, Identity, and Post-AIDS Discourse." *JAC* 24, No. 1 (January): 93–111.

Caron, David. 2001. *AIDS in French Culture: Social Ills, Literary Cures*. Madison: University of Wisconsin Press.

———. *My Father and I: The Marais and the Queerness of Community*. 2009. Ithaca: Cornell University Press.

———. *The Nearness of Others: Searching for Tact and Contact in the Age of HIV*. 2014. Minneapolis: University of Minnesota Press.

Davis, Oliver. 2015. "Leading by Example: A Queer Critique of Personalization and Coercive Community Governance in Act Up-Paris's Operation Against the Bareback Writers." *Sexualities* 18 (1/2): 141–57.

Dowsett, Gary W. 2017. "Abjection. Objection. Subjection: Rethinking the History of AIDS in Australian Gay Men's Futures." *Culture, Health, & Sexuality* 19, No. 9 (September): 935–47.

Dustan, Guillaume. [1996] 2013. *Dans ma chambre*. Paris: P.O.L.

———. *In My Room*. 1998. Trans. by Brad Rumph. London: Serpent's Tail.

———. *Je sors ce soir*. [1997] 2013. Paris: P.O.L.

Enault, Raffaël. 2018. *Dustan Superstar.* Paris: Éditions Robert Laffont.

Guibert, Hervé. 1990. *À l'ami qui ne m'a pas sauvé la vie*. Paris: Éditions Gallimard..

———. 1991. *Le protocole compassionnel*. Paris: Éditions Gallimard.

———. 1993. *The Compassion Protocol*. Trans. by James Kirkup. London: Quartet Books.

———. 1991. *To the Friend Who Did Not Save My Life*. Translated by Linda Coverdale. New York: Macmillan Publishing Company.

Kagan, Dion. 2018. *Positive Images: Gay Men and HIV/AIDS in the Culture of "Post-Crisis*." London: Bloomsbury.

Merriam-Webster, s.v. "raw," accessed October 5, 2018, http://www.merriam-webster.com/dictionary/raw.

———. "ghetto," accessed October 5, 2018, http://www.merriam-webster.com/dictionary/ghetto.

Pearl, Monica B. 2012. *AIDS Literature and Gay Identity: The Literature of Loss*. New York: Routledge.

Petrus, John. 2019. "Discussing the Undiscussable: Reflecting on the 'End' of 'AIDS.'" GLQ 25, No.1 (January): 67–72.

Poulin-Detour, William J. 2004. "French Gay Activism and the American Referent in Contemporary France." *The French Review* 78, No.1 (October): 118–25.

Pratt, Murray. 2012. "Getting it from Noise and Other Myths: AIDS and Intellectuals in France." *Paragraph* 35, No. 2: 181–96.

Race, Kane. 2009. *Pleasure Consuming Medicine: The Queer Politics of Drugs*. Durham: Duke University Press.

———. 2001. "The Undetectable Crisis: Changing Technologies of Risk." *Sexualities* 4, No.2 (2001): 167–89.

Rofes, Eric E. 1998. *Dry Bones Breathe: Gay Men Creating Post-AIDS Identities and Cultures.* Philadelphia: Haworth Press.

Tougaw, Jason. 2002. "Testimony and the Subjects of AIDS Memoirs." In *Extremities: Trauma, Testimony, and Community*, edited by Nancy Miller & Jason Tougaw, 165–185. University of Illinois Press.

Woubshet, Dagmawi. 2015. *The Calendar of Loss: Race, Sexuality, and Mourning in the Early Era of AIDS.* Baltimore: John Hopkins University Press.

NOTES

1. For a thorough examination of the epistemology of "Post-AIDS," see: Paul Butler, "Embracing AIDS: History, Identity, and Post-AIDS Discourse," *JAC* 24, no.1 (January 2004): 93–111. Gary W. Dowsett, "Abjection. Objection. Subjection: Rethinking the History of AIDS in Australian Gay Men's Futures," *Culture, Health, & Sexuality* 19, no. 9 (September 2017): 935–47. Dion Kagan, *Positive Images: Gay Men and HIV/AIDS in the Culture of "Post-Crisis"* (London: Bloomsbury, 2018). John Petrus, "Discussing the Undiscussable: Reflecting on the 'End' of 'AIDS,' GLQ 25, no.1 (January 2019): 67–72. Kane Race, *Pleasure Consuming Medicine: The*

Queer Politics of Drugs (Durham: Duke University Press, 2009), "The Undetectable Crisis: Changing Technologies of Risk," *Sexualities* 4, no.2 (2001): 167–89. Eric E. Rofes, *Dry Bones Breathe: Gay Men Creating Post-AIDS Identities and Cultures* (Philadelphia: Haworth Press, 1998).

2. For further reading on the prevailing scholarship concerning the role of French Universalism in the AIDS crisis, see: James N. Agar, "Queer in France: AIDS Disidentification in France," in *Queer in Europe: Contemporary Case Studies*, ed. Robert Gillett & Lisa Downing (London: Routledge, 2011), 57–70. Michal J. Bosia, "'Assassin!' AIDS and Neoliberal Reform in France," *New Political Science* 27, no. 3 (August 2006): 291–308. Jean-Pierre Boulé, *HIV Stories: The Archaeology of AIDS Writing in France* (Liverpool: Liverpool University Press, 2002). David Caron, *AIDS in French Culture: Social Ills, Literary Cures* (Madison: University of Wisconsin Press, 2001), *My Father and I: The Marais and the Queerness of Community* (Ithaca: Cornell University Press, 2009), *The Nearness of Others: Searching for Tact and Contact in the Age of HIV* (Minneapolis: University of Minnesota Press, 2014). William J. Poulin-Detour, "French Gay Activism and the American Referent in Contemporary France," *The French Review* 78, no. 1 (October 2004): 118–25. Murray Pratt, "Getting it from Noise and Other Myths: AIDS and Intellectuals in France," *Paragraph* 35, no. 2 (2012): 181–96.

3. For a thorough analysis of Act-Up Paris and their attacks on the bareback writers, see: Christophe Broqua, *Action=Vie: A History of AIDS Activism and Gay Politics in France*, trans. Jean-Yves Bart & Kel Pero (Philadelphia: Temple University Press, 2020).

4. The auto-da-fé-esque protest of Act-Up Paris was called "Abîmons les livres," roughly translated as "Let's spoil the books." For more, see: Oliver Davis, "Leading by Example: A Queer Critique of Personalization and Coercive Community Governance in Act-Up Paris's Operation Against the Bareback Writers," *Sexualities* 18 (1/2) (2015): 141–57.

5. Dustan's exclusion from the French literary canon as opposed to the more popularly known Guibert speaks volumes about the difference between the two authors' literature. It is not that one is queerer than the other, but Dustan's affinity for American culture and the English language, which distinctly separates him from Guibert and is well documented in his biography as well as his writing wherein he uses Anglicisms, references fashion labels, porn stars, music, etc. would disqualify him as being "French" enough to be included in the highly regulated world of French literature.

6. Further translations will be my own.

7. The entry for the word states: "A foundry for cannons was once located on an island that forms part of Venice, where in 1516 the Venetians restricted Jewish residence. The word *ghèto* became the name for the area and was borrowed into standard Italian as *ghetto*, with the meaning of 'section of a city where Jews are forced to live'" (emphasis in original).

Chapter Three

Kindling Kinships

Sexual Citizenship and Queer Constructions of Masculinity in the Works of Erik Rémès

Daniel N. Maroun

Erik Rémès, a trained clinical psychoanalyst, ruffled literary feathers when he published *Je bande donc je suis* [*I Get Hard Therefore I Am*] in 1999. The novel investigates the life of a serial barebacker and his sexual extremes. The premise of his work is predicated on a sex act, one that is repeated over and over again in the novel with each partner he shares. For Rémès, desire, sexuality, and AIDS are all a part of a longer 20th-century narrative that parallels its sexual evolution: "Peut-on parler du désir à la fin du vingtième siècle sans parler de sexualité donc de sida?" ["At the end of the twentieth-century, can we talk about desire without talking about sexuality and thus AIDS?"] (1999, 123). AIDS becomes a unique component of homosexuality in Rémès's texts because all action in the novel revolves around forms of condomless sexual acts that he has inscribed onto his very existence.[1] In doing so, he ties sex, sexuality, homosexuality to Frenchness right from the title of his first novel. He encodes sexuality and seropositivity onto his rewriting of the Cartesian *cogito* thus underscoring how important both the act and the serostatus truly are to *being*. In both *Je bande donc je suis* and *Serial Fucker,* Rémès constructs an HIV-positive masculinity through a ritualistic performance of barebacking that rejects a republican model of sexual citizenship. This performance of masculinity anchors itself in a repetitious act, that of a raw concept of seed spreading, a queer version of virility that aides in defining French models of gay sexual citizenship. This process of seroconversion repopulates his literary worlds and establishes a queer lineage, a bloodline that simulates heterosexual concepts of *filiation*. This interpretive strategy affords a new look at how seropositivity becomes a hallmark trait of Rémès's queer French Republic and empowers HIV-positive men to reclaim their sexual citizenship despite dominant Republican models that seek to neutralize the threat of "unsafe sex" and serotransmission.

BAREBACKING AND THE FUTURE OF QUEER REPRODUCTION

Reproduction and repopulation as critical concepts in Rémès's oeuvre sit at a unique intersection of Lee Edelman's "no futurity" and José Esteban Muñoz's queer sociality. In *No Future* (2004), Edelman transvalues the claim that queerness has no inherent value in the future because homosexuals lack the inherent inability to reproduce; that society is dominated by an imperative of "reproductive futurism" where the child is a political entity (2004, 3). Edelman then explores what the theoretical and ethical implications would be in a world that rejected the child as the crux of futurity. He argues against the notion that queerness needs to be anchored toward a futurity because such an anticipatory gesture of hopefulness continues to posit "queer" as nonrealizable. One can contend that bareback sex and seroconversion are somewhat future-oriented in that the transmission of the disease ensures its future; however, I suggest that Rémès's depiction of bareback sex and those who engage in it align more with Edelman's notion of the "sinthomosexual," a figure who incarnates Lacan's definition of the death drive (35). The sinthomosexual destroys the symbolic universe to ensure the survival of itself as the subject which I interpret as Rémès undoing the French Republican knots that tie down definitions of (queer) sexual citizenship.

Additionally, I argue that Rémès's acts of seroconversion are not embedded in futurity of the disease, but instead in terms of positionality and sociality. Barebacking is rooted in a deliberate performance of transmission that aligns more with Muñoz's model of queer futurity/sociability. Seroconversion is an act of resistance that Rémès's protagonist Berlin Tintin promotes. Muñoz argues that "queerness is essentially about the rejection of a here and now and an insistence on potentiality" (2019, 1). Rémès rejects the essentialism of heteronormativity and seronegativity, which I propose are the "here and now" that Muñoz discusses, by emphasizing the potentiality that barebacking consigns to existence. For Muñoz, queer futurity is a utopian impulse embedded in queer collectivity, a hope that new ways of belonging and existence are just over the "queer horizon"(20). Queer futurity depends on potentiality as well as a resistance to an anxious present. For Rémès, this potentiality is the signification of bareback sex and the resistance to dominant safe sex and heteronormative discourses that have used condoms as physical and symbolic barriers to protect against the clinical and "moral danger attributed to gay sexual pleasure" (Race 2015). However, bareback sex is not merely performative; seropositivity and the act of seroconversion in *Je bande* concretize queer sexual citizenship for the individuals participating in it because queer sexual citizenship is inconcomitant with the French universalist model. Barebacking hence affords a plurality of possible futures, of futures that are collective and based in an aspiration of sero-normativity.

The concept of sexual citizenship is a unique interpretative strategy for queer communities as it bridges the public and private spheres—two very discordant entities in French culture. Popularized by David T. Evans in his *Sexual Citizenship: The Material Construction of Sexualities* (1993), the term has come to embody the political and cultural implications that expressions of sexuality can have. This term is of fastidious interest when studying French HIV/AIDS narratives as it legitimizes their expression of masculinity, their subculture, and their sufferance when compared to the dominating narratives of French republicanism and universalism. In short, the principle of sexual citizenship permits marginalized sexualities or genders to confront the public with the private. It also provides the seropositive gay community the ability to structure new performances of what masculinity is. Butler's notion of performativity is vital to understanding how Rémès and other HIV/AIDS writers (de)construct masculinity insofar as she purports that gender is culturally constructed through stylized acts in a given epoch and that these acts are repeated (1990, 144). I understand performativity as an act that constitutes the subject through public, repetitious rituals and therefore will argue that gay seropositive masculinity is indeed stylized through a repetitious act of seroconversion. Reproduction need not be strictly biological, but it can also be "social" as R.W. Connell maintains (2005, 73).

HIV/AIDS is intrinsically tied to discussions of masculinity, especially homosexual performances of masculinity, because the initial onset of the epidemic was viewed as fate, a consequence of homosexuality, a manifestation of sins that defied all biomedical knowledge and targeted a subset of the population. The disease clashes/ed with Western concepts of gender norms and notions of sexuality as it was an attack on all forms of normativity, the most theoretical of which was the concept that it dismantled the body's immunological response to defend itself much like homosexuality deconstructs sociosexual norms. By seeming to only target the gay population, the French response lagged as it battled negotiating a community's needs and its own universalist principles.[2] French universalism privileges/d the heteronormative model under the guise of equality but in doing so only isolated the marginalized further. Critics Best and Crowley conclude that authors like Rémès and Guillaume Dustan who celebrated seropositive barebacking behavior created an "identitarian position" pitted against that of French universalism and republicanism. Best and Crowley also argue further that the "emphatic celebration of anal pleasure (i.e., sex) it entails, constitutes a defiant rejection of universalism dismissed as merely a cover for the propagation of familial, reproductive heteronormativity" (2007, 89). The dismissal of France's core republican principle portends a radical threat which subverts normative discourses on sexuality only motivating an author like Rémès to destabilize the universalist principle further. The subculture of barebacking inside these novels supplants universalism with seropositivity thus allowing participants to ignore French republicanism and adopt a *barebackinism* founded on queerness.

THE INTENTIONS OF BAREBACKING

The definition of the term "bareback" carries an intentionality with it: an intentionality to have unprotected sex, an intentionality to possibly seroconvert someone, and an intentionality to possibly be seroconverted, all of which convey an implicit "risk" acknowledged by those participating in bareback sex (Carballo-Diéguez et al. 2010). Barebacking also connotes a masculine performativity since the term echoes a cowboy's riding without a saddle. Cowboys can be lawless vigilantes commonly living outside the norms; those who use the term "bareback" and engage in it reappropriate an idealized masculinity—someone willing to take risks. Bareback sex thus is a queer performance of masculinity. It is a sexual practice that has long been associated with the queer community even before and surely during the epidemic (Florêncio 2020, 3). The actions of Berlin Tintin, Rémès's autofictional alter-ego in *Je bande*, belong to a group of gay men who have discovered that on the basis of viral transmission or serostatus they can form a kinship, a network of relationships that resemble heteronormative familial bonds. However, the reappropriation of these heteronormative familial features run the risk of reproducing exactly what this queering gesture of seroconversion seeks to erase. I would argue that while this reappropriation of the familial is a theoretical risk, it is still a queer version of a normative relationship. Heteronormative families and kin are tied together by blood much like the bonds that the protagonist inside Rémès's novels *Serial Fucker* and *Je bande donc je suis* share through serostatus. Instead of sharing genetic resemblance, these men share immunological resemblance. This shared similitude gives meaning to the subculture, a *raison d'être* that establishes their community. However, a large portion of critical commentary on bareback sex treats it like a "pathological behavior" (Dean 2009, 9; 48), and any other interpretation would promote an egregious lifestyle that goes against the grain of society aiding the disease and preventing its morally just and future elimination. Sadly, this point of view does nothing to explain the reason why barebacking occurs. Rather, it continues to label condomless sex as a disorder that promotes the spread of a life-threatening disease. This stance prevents us from interrogating the bonds of kinship that created this culture and unified it in the face of legal, cultural, and medical challenges that wanted to eliminate it in the '90s. Tim Dean in *Unlimited Intimacy* argues that in order to understand barebacking, we need to treat it like any culture/group/community and approach it anthropologically, gaining insight into its language, rites, traditions, and mores. This disciplinary approach undoubtedly unveils much about a group; however, examining barebacking through this anthropological lens may relegate the action to a select group of individuals rather than a broader, cultural queer praxis of condomless sex. Instead of moralizing bareback sex, reading Rémès's novels tenders the ability to interrogate the bonds of kinship that are created through barebacking and serotransmission. His defense and valorization of bareback sex, alongside the more notable Guillaume Dustan, confounded and upset activist associations like Act-Up Paris who promoted a certain responsibility among same-sex partners, defining barebacking as an "ideology of risk taking" (Broqua 2020, 233). By creating a moral ideology, Act-Up was able to create a sociosexual enemy that society could label the enemy. It is important to note what is at stake here when Rémès promotes condomless sex. He is not suggesting being irresponsible, but rather he is promoting the plurality of desire and pleasure of which barebacking is one. Rémès's writing represents "plus qu'une simple apologie de *bareback.* Voir dans ses œuvres une pure défense des pratiques sexuelles non protégées serait reléguer aux oubliettes la part de nuance qu'il tente d'introduire" ["more than a simple apology of barebacking. To see, in his works, a pure defense of unprotected sexual practices would be to cast any nuance that he is attempting to introduce into obscurity"] which suggests that he is paving the way for a variety of peripheral sexual practices (Najm 2016, 119). Additionally, bareback sex creates consanguinity among the men engaging in this action that negates the need for women. Men reproduce among themselves, physically sharing their bodily fluids and genetic material to breed a new progeny made in the essence of the seeder. The works included in this section will demonstrate how the protagonists' contaminated seed breeds new definitions of masculinity in a queer literary universe that reproduces via a viral transmission.

BAREBACKING AND EXISTENCE

Rémès's first novel *Je bande donc je suis* represents the candid diary of Berlin Tintin's exploits. The text is a *bildungsroman* of sexual acceptance that details life as a gay French man who is HIV positive. It chronicles the hero's journey from youth to adulthood, from shame to acceptance, from seronegativity to seropositivity. Berlin Tintin's psychological and moral growth parallels the extremity of his sexual pleasures as he grows to accept himself as a gay French man who pushes the boundaries of normative culture. *Je bande donc je suis* juxtaposes two worlds: heteronormativity and the "other." The novel emphasizes Berlin Tintin's journey from one of these worlds to the other as well as his emotional and psychological responses as he transgresses normative boundaries and rejects heterosexual hegemony. After his sexual initiation into the world, Tintin explores the impact of his homosexuality and future seropositivity writing: "Ce fut l'accès la toute première fois. L'accès au logos, à l'existence" ["This was access for the very first time. Access to the *logos*, to existence"] (Rémès 1999, 23). Additionally, his initiation to the sexual world comes from the "other" since the man with whom he has his first sexual encounter is an Arab, a socioethnically marked "other" in the French context. In other words, his abandonment of heterosexuality is accessed through the "other."

Barebacking proposes a solution, a way to broker social exile and French republicanism by means of a new negotiation of sexual citizenship. Thus, Rémès constructs masculinity around seroconversion establishing a community that shares a bloodline that is passed down from one man to another through seroconversion. Additionally, sexual exchanges are not the only way in which Rémès establishes a change; it is also through the reading of his text and the readers themselves. The act of reading HIV/AIDS narratives becomes "high-risk" because this behavior can "threaten the plenitude of both the supposedly healthy subject and its discourse" as Caron has argued in the past (2001, 138). The reader is brought into this ritual in a very Barthesian *scriptible* fashion when the Rémèsian narrator claims: "Comment provoquer en lui le désir de lire, voire d'en jouir?" ["How do I provoke in them the desire to read, even to get off"] (Rémès 1999, 74). Reading is equated to fucking in Rémès's text quite similarly to how reading and fucking are positioned in the works of acclaimed author Hervé Guibert. Rémès's narrative contains a laundry list of sexual exchanges with various, anonymous partners, but the greatest one of all is not listed because it happens at the time of reading. Reading thus does not remain an intellectual act but a physiological one as well. By flipping the role of the reader, he recodes his text from a place where the pleasure is simply in the act of reading about Berlin Tintin's conversion and escapades—a *lisible* (or legible) text. Rémès's perversion of Cartesian logic of "je bande donc je suis" ["I get hard therefore I am"] is further transformed into "Il bande, donc nous sommes" ["He gets hard therefore we are"], for our participation in the text is based on Tintin's sexuality. Furthermore, the *writability* of the text is enhanced if one engages the reader as the actor and rescripts Tintin's adage to "Nous bandons donc il est" ["We get hard therefore he is"], which is to say that our textual jouissance is what creates Tintin's textual existence. This concept is crucial because it is not only the actions of the protagonist that establish a queer HIV-positive performativity of masculinity but also the act of reading which furthers Berlin Tintin's goal of populating a seropositive Republic.

LIFE AND DEATH

Tintin's seroconversion in this novel plays a dichotomous role dividing life and death. The former plays a central part as his seroconversion marks both an end and a beginning: "Pourtant après mon hécatombe virale, je ne pensais plus pouvoir ressentir une quelconque satisfaction" ["However, after my viral disaster, I didn't think I was able to feel any satisfaction anymore"] (58). Tintin's seroconversion becomes a sacrifice from which he ultimately gains something. He inscribes death onto his HIV status not solely because it is medically justifiable, but also because it marks the end of a former heterosexual reality that relegated his sexuality to the periphery. When analyzing Cyril Collard's depiction of a gay Paris in *Les Nuits Fauves*, Lawrence Schehr argues that AIDS is personified as death but metonymized in anonymous sex—I suggest that for Rémès's novels AIDS is metonymized in bareback sex (Schehr 2009). Tintin wants to metaphorically end his life to be reborn as positive: "Je savais dès le début qu'un jour je mettrais fin à tout cela, à cette vie-là, pour en recommencer une autre, une toute nouvelle vie, belle et fraîche" ["I knew from the get go that I would end all of this, this life, to start another one, entirely knew, beautiful, fresh"] (Rémès 1999, 59). Tintin erases his past and creates a constant positivity, a constant presence of AIDS where there is no literary "before." In *Serial Fucker*, Rémès echoes the same sentiment regarding a new life that AIDS has given him: "Moi, j'aimerais plutôt m'inscrire dans une histoire positive de la renaissance. De la résurrection même" ["Me, I would rather inscribe myself in a positive history of rebirth. Of resurrection even"] (192). For Tintin, his seroconversion is life. Rémès's equivocation of seropositivity as life is even more meaningful when juxtaposed against the scathing attacks he publically suffered from Didier Lestrade, founder of Act-Up Paris, who regularly depicted unprotected intercourse as murder (Broqua 2020, 221). Rémès is essentially rejecting ideological moralization and role modeling how condomless sex is life.

Life and death thus become a leitmotif in the novel, on one hand due to the obvious medical and physical implications of HIV/AIDS, and on the other because it creates the necessary background for Rémès to explore a sero-positive masculinity. One can argue that life for Tintin did not start until he was HIV positive. More crucial for this *roman d'apprentissage*, his pre-HIV life preceded his journey because the virus is the indicator of change: "Ma séropositivité a provoqué une remise en question profonde, mais, là encore, belle dans son carnage" ["My seropositivity provoked a deep question but even there, still, it was beautiful in its carnage"] (1999, 62). Therefore, death becomes a precursor to seropositivity, and in Rémès's novel cultural logic is reversed; seronegativity inhabits the role of death while seropositivity embodies life, a birth that allows for a new exploration of vitality. Death becomes a sexual impetus as bareback sex and seroconversion forge the possibility of new life. HIV/AIDS is synonymous with death, and death drives Berlin Tintin to the extremes of sexual practice: [L]a mort c'est excitant. La mort fait bander, la mort fait jouir" ["Death is sexy. Death gets you hard, death gets you off"] (109).

Rémès takes control of death, claiming ownership over it so that he can dictate its meaning. This act of control is how he finds so much pleasure in it: "Après tout, être condamné à mourir, c'est être condamné à vivre, donc à jouir" ["After all, to be condemned to death is to be condemned to live, thus to cum"] (58). He continues to associate death with sex and sex with life. Sex, life, and death blend into one and lose their natural opposition. They all ultimately bring the reader back to the title of the work, *Je bande donc je suis*. There is no escaping the sexual nature of both HIV/AIDS and the queerness that Rémès promotes in his novels since physical *jouissance* is predicated on life, and life, ironically, is predicated on death which is metonymized by seropositivity. Life and death mingle more in an S&M scene from the novel. Some friends take Tintin to a brothel for an S&M night "chez les zéteros" ["with the straights"] where he relishes the chance to push the limits of normative sexuality. He and his women friends become aggressors and active partners, flipping gender roles. His girlfriend Malicia "fiste Jean-Luc Eurostar à deux mains devant un parterre de zétéros abasourdis" ["fists Jean-Luc Eurostar with two hands in front of a stunned audience of breeders"] while he and his other girlfriend Metale "latte[nt] la gueule à un esclave hétéro" ["whips the mug of a straight sub"] (108). This sexual role reversal allows the previously marginalized (women and gay men) to dominate the sexual encounter much to the amazement and bewilderment of the straight onlookers. Their supremacy is unhinged in this scene as peripheral sexual practices take main stage. Their final dismissal comes from Tintin: "un bon

quelqu'un qui n'a pas honte de ses opinions et de son caractère et de ses caractéristiques" ["Someone who accepts himself . . . that's someone who isn't ashamed of his opinions of his character and his behaviors"] (2007, 112). This viewpoint is one that is further reiterated by Sandrine, another interviewee, who states that "'S'assumer' veut dire être bien dans la tête, dans sa sexualité et vivre normalement" ["'s'assumer' means to feel good about yourself, about your sexuality and to live normally"] (112). This French process not only strikes a unique contrast to the dualism of the American expression being "in" or "out" of the closet but also with how Tintin cannot resolve French cultural reality of the nineties with the seropositive world he creates in the novel. Nevertheless, his insistence on accepting himself foreshadows the trajectory the novel takes and juxtaposes shame with acceptance by the end: "J'ai aimé assumer ma vie . . . J'ai aimé mon virus . . . J'ai aimé la vie, ce qu'elle m'a donné, ce qu'elle me donnera encore" ["I loved being comfortable with my life . . . I loved my virus . . . I loved life, what it gave me, what still has to give me"] (Rémès 1999, 239). Rémès's text illustrates the *roman d'apprentissage* of a youngster going out into the world to seek his fortune by juxtaposing his early naiveté and shame of the queer world with his expertise and fulfillment by the end: "Je ne regrette rien. J'aimerai toujours la vie" ["I don't regret anything. I will always love life"] (239). In doing so, Rémès reaffirms Tintin's trajectory and masculine affirmation as the character constructs himself through sex acts, asserting new queer models of masculinity.

This queer seropositive model of masculinity evolves to mimic heterosexual notions of kinship and democracy therein by establishing a homosexual concept of *filiation* where the ties are not intergenerational genetics but sero-genetics, and the representation is not communitarian but socially equal. The bareback norms in Rémès's text parody heterosexual filiation whose bloodline is secured by purposeful transmission. By engaging in the intentionality of bareback sex, Tintin belongs to this "group" or "kin." He is initiated into this tribe. From the early stages of his conversion, Tintin knows he is a part of something bigger, an obligation to explore and expand the queer universe of the novel: "Car je sais bien que cette mise en abîme de mon être portera un jour ses fruits" ["Thus I know well that this story within a story of my being will bear its fruit one day"] (59). The fruit of his seed is the seroconverted offspring now virally connected. Rémès' texts create a biological necessity wherein seropositive semen establishes a new generation of seroconverts. In *Serial Fucker,* the narrator humorously discusses how "les députés de droite" ["Right-wing congressmen"] want to outlaw "l'insémination du Sida" ["the insemination of AIDS"] (2005, 9–10). Insemination is broadly defined as the biological process of introducing sperm into female reproductive organs with the purpose of reproduction. Rémès's reappropriation of insemination and barebacking for biological purposes replaces biological reproduction with seroreproduction. Rémès is negotiating a queer masculinity that involves a futurity, a futurity that is based in sociality as Muñoz would elaborate. Most interesting is the emphasis on ejaculate, his viral seed, that Rémès creates which frames a new queer aesthetic (Lee 2014). Instead of reifying a sacred masculinity but between men, Rémès is introducing quite literally a *toxic* masculinity that is grounded in serotransmission.

LINEAGE AND LEGACY

Serial Fucker shares a similar reproductive narrative that is built in *Je bande*; however, the narration is more autofictive with a larger presence of "je" ["I"] telling the story instead of a narrator discussing Tintin. The reader subsequently confronts Rémès's own story rather than have it transformed into the sexual escapades of Berlin Tintin as in *Je bande.* Insemination, as stated in *Serial Fucker,* does not associate with HIV/AIDS discourses typically, but its infiltration into this novel reinforces the classical gender role and function of masculinity prescribed in these non-normative novels. For Rémès, insemination allows for the spreading of the virus so that it becomes the communal trait passed on like ancestral genes from generation to generation, or orgy to orgy in this case. The tribe creates a bloodline that becomes intimately linked to any discussion on HIV/AIDS since the disease is epidemiologically attached to all hemotransfusions. Blood becomes sacred in this community as Tintin seeks to establish progeny that will continue his legacy, his lineage: "Alors, je continuais imperturbable, ma quête phallique du Saint-Graal" ["Thus I continued imperturbably my phallic quest for the Holy Grail"] (1999, 59). The allusion to the holy blood of Christ coagulates the importance that seroconversion has in the novel and for the bareback community. The transubstantiation of wine to blood in Christianity allows followers to imbibe the blood of Christ, to consume him in an attempt to seek redemption. Each time the wine is consumed, it is an act of remembrance that reinscribes Christ's death ("Do this in memory of me"). Seroconversion slightly mimics the process as blood is transubstantiated into the blood of HIV life, and each seroconversion reiterates Rémès's initial conversion. By passing on the virus, the narrator is in theory asking his partners to also "Do this in memory of me." Additionally, it is worth observing the common but false etymology of Saint-Graal as *sangréal*, a term that further underlines the concept of a royal bloodline that is preserved and passed down from one "asshole" to the next, as Rémès narrates (59).

The entire bareback community is a "cocktail à base de sang et de sperme" ["a cocktail made from blood and sperm"] (2005, 217), a mixture where blood represents the genealogical link and sperm the necessary element of creation and seeding. It is the condomless aspect of the bareback community, its lack of protection or rawness as it pre-dates pre- and post-prophylactics that affords itself this opportunity of transmission and thus establishing a family. Subsequently, it is this very family unit that Rémès's novels structure and promote. There is no question that seroconcordance in the bareback community is the tying bond. At a bareback orgy during Christmas, the narrator gazes at the men around him, noting: "Nous étions toutes des grosses putes assoiffées de suc, membres de la même famille, unis par le même feu, brûlant de souche commune. Un lien de sperme et de sang, indéfectible" ["We all were these giant whores thirsty for the juice, members of the same family, united by the same fire, burning with common origins. A union of unfailing semen and blood"] (12). The transfer of serostatus from a positive to a negative revitalizes the notion of transfiliation—but what is transferred is not simply an anthropological relationship and codified normativity, it is also a genealogy of sufferance for a community.[3] The concept of transfiliation becomes even more profound when we view it from the lens of readership: Rémès's novels are purchased, read, shared, discussed which creates another community that *transmits his seropositvity.*

It is therefore through this queered family unit that Rémès reclaims and constructs masculinity and builds a futurity. Rémèsian masculinity is based on the sex act of bareback and the potentiality of seroconversion. The latter then becomes the referent for the Rémès's bareback community as even Rémès toys with the concept of his community replacing families and condomless orgies replacing family gatherings: "Ce meeting [orgie], c'est une vraie réunion de famille" ["This meeting [orgy], is a real family reunion"] (1999, 83), where specific sexual pleasures (fellatio, fisting, penetration, etc.) replace traditional bonding activities like fishing, football, or board games. Rémès's Tintin abandons the futurity of children and fully adopts the queer sociality of serokinship. The queer family supplants the traditional family model and becomes the main source of homocultural norms like barebacking and potentially even more extreme forms of sexual practice.

It is important to revisit two key concepts mentioned earlier: Republican duty and *assumer son identité* ["to accept one's identity"]. French republicanism idolizes a social contract that engages the citizen directly with the government. Such an ideology requires a heteronormative family unit to promote it, and thus populating the Republic with law-abiding citizens becomes paramount to success through conscripts who "assume" their obligation. Viral transmission queers the notion of the French republic because the "child" as Edelman asserted earlier, is no longer its future—the seroconvert becomes the horizon of futurity. The narrator realizes the need for a sero-procreation and promotes condomless sex: "Je suis pour la libre circulation du virus" ["I am for the free circulation of the virus"] (110)—a neomarxist approach that commodifies the virus as a market good that individuals can purchase or exchange. Tintin in *Je bande* buys into this commodification of the body and upholds his sero-republican duty of infecting others—populating his literary universe: "Berlin Tintin ne les comptait plus ceux qu'il avait maintenant contaminés. Et un et deux et trois: sida! Ainsi Tintin agrandissait la grande famille des sidéens" ["Berlin Tintin no longer kept count of those whom he had contaminated. And one, and two, and three: AIDS! Thus Tintin grew his family of PWA"] (115). He posits himself as an alpha male breeder, a Genghis Khan of sorts, adopting his duty to procreate *à la seropo*.[4] His use of "et un, et deux, et trois: sida!" echoes the 1998 World Cup French win against Brazil. France's participation in the World Cup can be viewed as a republican moment of the country coming together; here Rémès queers that model so that the nation comes together for AIDS.

Tintin continues his narrative diatribe adding: "Les corps se suivent et se ressemblent, s'enchâssent, s'assemblent, s'emboîtent, et s'encastrent" ["The bodies are all lined up, look the same, set in their place, gathered, interlocked, embedded one after the other"] (85), a quote in which I argue the use of the pronominal verb stresses the reciprocal nature of serotransmission among those engaging in bareback sex. Moreover, the choice of verbs paints a vivid picture of bodies-as-pieces arranged in a perfect puzzle epitomizing corporality. This compartmentalization of the body echoes João Florêncio's argument of how Rémès's text, in part, subverts Western thought of a unified body, allowing for a more porous and permeable iteration of masculinity to be performed (2020, 62–63). However, this compartmentalization has a literary lineage as David Caron points out that HIV/AIDS author Hervé Guibert was "obsessed with the dissolution of the body" in turn allowing him to explore AIDS more thematically (2001, 117).

The promotion of safe sex prevents sero-procreation but also undermines classical notions of masculinity. Dean explains that safe sex emasculates gay men by removing the "risk" these men are naturally inclined to take: "The prophylaxis afforded by condoms is reserved for those who can't handle the real thing. Rather than offering protection, condoms make a man and his masculinity vulnerable to doubt or derision" (2009, 53). The protection condoms afford male individuals who engage in bareback sex ironically emasculates them; thus, barebacking reinforces classical structures of bravery and courage that are assigned to masculinity but from inside a queer model. Barebacking, seroconversion, and seropositivity remain intertwined in these two texts as the basis for existence and futurity. Tintin in *Je bande* and Rémès in *Serial Fucker* assert that existence is predicated on the presence of this virus. Take for example Tintin's claim, "Mon virus c'était la vie, seropo ergo sum" ["My virus was life, seropo ergo sum"] (Rémès 1999, 180). This claim is in stark contrast to HIV/AIDS novels of Hervé Guibert that bring to the fore suffering (*pathos*) and marginality. The presumed suffering that sociocultural institutions have imposed on people living with AIDS is transformed and reappropriated to represent a drive, a pulsion: "Il n'y a pas d'éros sans pathos" ["There is no eros without pathos"] (186). His construction of masculinity revolves around the disease: "Il m'a d'abord détruit et puis construit" ["It destroyed me first, then it built me back up"] (181), and his performance of said masculinity depends on serotransmission. His construction of an HIV-positive masculinity and the performance of it are entangled but dependent on one sole point—his seropositivity: "Je ne pouvais vivre sans mon pathos" ["I couldn't live without my pathos"] (179). His virus becomes his best and longest relationship—meaningful, fulfilling, and passionate, and its transmission grants a lineage of immortality.

These two novels showcase a reappropriation of sociomoral condemnation allowing for a new homonormative narrative to appear, centered on seropositivity. Rémès's two texts break away from Guibert's tradition of writing about life with the disease, assuming a new model of what can be done with the disease. In doing so, Rémès evades a discourse of discipline about this serostatus which allows him to control how his "truth" is structured. David Caron elaborates on this same utilitarian stance of the disease when he writes: "To share, in that sense, is a matter not of unveiling some kind of truth but of making and remaking knowledge together in order to serve our needs" (2014, 134). Rémès controls how the disease describes his life—it is a tool for his self-description that he uses to define himself.

By considering HIV/AIDS as an equally important descriptive category of Frenchness and queerness, Rémès gives equal space to how it affects identity construction, that is, sexual citizenship. This form of sexual citizenship transforms HIV/AIDS from a virus and a disease to a qualifying normative characteristic within the novel. It becomes a social construct that identifies its members. The virus becomes a genetic link that binds all barebackers together, their common trait passed on from partner to partner, mutating, shifting, and evolving along the way. This functionality of barebacking is a remarkable feat considering that anal intercourse and other non-vaginal, non-heterosexual forms of intercourse deny the value "of productivity, futurity and vitality conventionally symbolized by the act of heterosexual vaginal penetration" (Best and Crowley 2007, 84). By demystifying the reproductive model, Rémès breathes new life into the meaning of HIV/AIDS. Foucault argued that sexuality is about creating new possibilities, a possibility where Rémès shows how masculinity is reclaimed in a queer model of seroreproduction. Rémès is not arguing for liberation; he is arguing that his serostatus has meaning. For Foucault, extreme sexualities are a way to shift the teleological reproductive function of the genitals to one that is a locus of new possibilities, new sexualities, new sexual practices, and new identities (1978, 36).

Rémès's works, as well as those of his contemporary Guillaume Dustan, testify to the founding of a new sexual body that justifies extreme sexual practices. For both of these authors, sex is operative, a means by which they can transgress boundaries and perform queer iterations that reappropriate a masculinity. Such an interpretation adds to the critical body of work that views both Rémès and Dustan's sexual exploits and bareback promotion as a means of destabilizing heterocentric French society.[5] Indeed, their subversive act is destabilizing in nature—quinessentially queer. However, I additionally propose that analyzing the symbolic act of barebacking enables us to draw larger conclusions about the literary representation of HIV positive queer masculinities. To study masculinity through the lens of seropositivity is more meaningful when we admit that there is not a masculine referent inside of French seropositive literature. The manner in which these authors nuance masculinity is "in no way limited by the received knowledge of the past" (Schehr 2009, 75). Seropositivite masculinites are negotiated through this process of writing about their own positionality with AIDS.

A study of the representational meaning of barebacking in the novels of Erik Rémès is meaningful because of the snapshot it provides of what barebacking meant at this specific time when risks were much higher. Indeed, because of the advent of PrEP and PEP our attention should turn to what condomless sex means among gay men and their performativity of a queer masculinity. It begs us to wonder how the actions of Berlin Tintin in *Je bande* or those of the narrator in *Serial Fucker* would be received in a contemporary world where risk is controlled through pharmacological intervention. Perhaps that is the next phase of queer sexual performativity—how the chemical or pharmaceutical encourage or inhibit new queer masculinities and how modern antiretroviral drugs have embodied the biopolitics of self-care granting autonomy to "the autonomous neo-liberal consumer" (of sex) (Florêncio 2020, 6).

BIBLIOGRAPHY

Best, Victoria, and Martin Crowley. 2007. *The New Pornographies: Explicit Sex in Recent French Fiction and Film*. Manchester: Manchester University Press.

Broqua, Christophe. 2020. *Action=Vie: A History of AIDS Activism and Gay Politics in France*. Translated by Jean-Yves Bart and Kel Pero. Philadelphia: Temple University Press.

Carballo-Diéguez, Alex, Ana Ventuneac, and José Bauermeister. 2012. "'Bareback'—Definitions and Identity: Constructs' Limitation for HIV-Prevention Research." Essay. In *Routledge Handbook of Sexuality, Health and Rights*. London: Routledge.

Caron, David. 2001. *AIDS in French Culture: Social Ills, Literary Cures*. Madison, WI: University of Wisconsin Press.

———, David. 2014. *The Nearness of Others: Searching for Tact and Contact in the Age of HIV*. Minneapolis: University of Minnesota Press.

Edelman, Lee. 2004. *No Future Queer Theory and the Death Drive*. Durham: Duke University Press.

Evans, David. 2013. *Sexual Citizenship The Material Construction of Sexualities*. London: Taylor and Francis.

Florêncio, João. 2020. *Bareback Porn, Porous Masculinities, Queer Futures: the Ethics of Becoming-Pig*. Abingdon, Oxon: Routledge.

Foucault, Michel. 1978. *The History of Sexuality*. London: Penguin Classics.

Gunther, S. 2009. *Elastic Closet: a History of Homosexuality in France 1942-Present*. Palgrave Macmillan.

Lee, Byron. 2014. "It's a Question of Breeding: Visualizing Queer Masculinity in Bareback Pornography." *Sexualities* 17, no. 1–2: 100–120. https://doi.org/10.1177/1363460713511099.

Muñoz, José Esteban. 2019. *Cruising Utopia: the Then and There of Queer Futurity*. New York: New York University Press.

Najm, Daoud et al. 2016. "Défense et Illustration du Bareback: De la Responsabilité à l'oeuvre Chez Guillaume Dustan et Erik Rémès." Essay. In *Littérature Et Sida, Alors Et Encore*, 112–20. Leiden; Boston: Brill Rodopi.

Provencher, Denis M. 2007. *Queer French: Globalization, Language, and Sexual Citizenship in France*. London: Ashgate.

Race, Kane. 2015. "Reluctant Objects." *GLQ: A Journal of Lesbian and Gay Studies* 22, no. 1: 1–31. https://doi.org/10.1215/10642684-3315217.

Rémès, Erik. 1999. *Je Bande Donc Je Suis*. Paris: Balland.

———, Erik. 2005. *Serial Fucker: Journal D'un Barebacker: Roman*. Paris: Blanche.

Schehr, Lawrence R. 2009. "Fragmented Territories: AIDS and Paris in Les Nuits Fauves of Cyril Collard." *French Forum* 34, no. 1: 53–65. https://doi.org/10.1353/frf.0.0073.

———, Lawrence R. 2009. *French Postmodern Masculinities: From Neuromatrices to Seropositivity*. Liverpool: Liverpool University Press.

———, Lawrence R. 2004. "Reading Serial Sex: The Case of Erik Rémès." *L'Esprit Créateur* 44, no. 3: 94–104. https://doi.org/10.1353/esp.2010.0256.

NOTES

1. See Lawrence Schehr "Reading Serial Sex: The Case of Erik Rémès" *L'Esprit Créateur* (2004).

2. See David Caron, *AIDS in French Culture: Social Ills, Literary Cures,* (Wisconsin: University of Wisconsin Press, 2001: 42, 283) as well as Scott Gunther, *The Elastic Closet,* (New York: Palgrave MacMillian, 2008: 79–80).

3. *Serial Fucker* differs from *Je bande* in that there is no moment of seroconversion. In *Serial Fucker* the narrator is always HIV-positive thus normalizing the

serostatus from the start and marginalizing anything else. The periphery becomes the center for the entire novel.

4. It is worth noting how Rémès tabulates those individuals he has seroconverted or shared in their conversion process through the epistrophe of "Le sida, aux suivants" (*Serial Fucker* 59, 97, 99, 115, 119, 120), a record of his mission.

5. See James S. William, "Resurrecting Cocteau: Gay (In)visibility and the Clean-up of French Culture," *Modern and Contemporary France* (2006), 317–330; and Hugues Marchal, "Chroniques de la vie sexuelle" *Le Nouveau Magazine Littéraire* (2003).

Chapter Four

Covering Up

Condomless Sex, (Ir)responsibility, and Risk in France

Brian Troth

For Riley Snorton, "Crisis begets more crises" (2020, 316). At the peak of the AIDS epidemic in 1994, gay men found themselves embroiled in a medical crisis as well as an *ethical* one. Certain sexual practices have always been considered taboo: anal sex, sex among men, and extramarital sex. What differs here is that sex at the height of a deadly epidemic that is spread through contact with bodily fluids carries the weight of what it means to be *responsible*. Specifically, inasmuch as a crisis "is an occasion for judgment, an opportunity to render power," a crisis is a call to redefine what constitutes responsible behavior (Cheng et al. 2020, 1). We can understand how a society defines responsibility at any given moment through the judgments that it makes on certain behaviors. It is an unfortunate reality for marginalized people that it is more attractive to "sympathize more with the murderous 'moral' fury" than with those most affected by HIV/AIDS (Bersani 1987, 201). In my contribution to this volume on rawness, I propose an analysis of Erik Rémès's corpus alongside more contemporary representations of risk to show the ways in which transgressive sexual practices allow us to reconsider how we define risky behavior, responsible practices, and the processes by which we protect ourselves. I have chosen to temper this analysis with the inclusion of public health campaigns which, by their very public nature, expose how risk is portrayed in the public sphere.

A RELIGION OF RISK-TAKING

Let us first consider the two versions of Act Up-Paris's campaign "Baiser sans capote ça vous fait jouir?" ["Does Condomless Sex Make You Come?"]. The campaign images were released for Gay Pride on June 26, 1999, and later released online in July 1999. The two posters are visually quite similar.[1] They each consisted of one black-and-white photo, explicitly depicting sexual acts between men and clearly evoking the exchange of bodily fluids between two sexual partners. In one, a man is delivering oral sex to a man who is ejaculating on the former. In the other, the camera frames an uncovered penis in closeup as it enters another man's anus. The caption on both versions asks if unprotected sex makes the viewer climax. The use of "vous" ["you"] directly speaks to the audience, pointing a finger toward the reader and imploring them to evaluate their sexual practices. The images are offset by large chunks of text that feature identical lists of reasons why the viewer may be tempted to engage in unprotected sex. Among them: public health campaigns are not targeting HIV/AIDS, and antiretroviral treatments offer relief from the fear that the disease is fatal. The campaign's imagery frames a certain rawness that guides this chapter. The condomless penetration depicts a raw act of sexuality, further reinforced by the explicit nature of the images. By emphasizing the rawness of condomless sex, the campaign establishes unprotected sex as a "religion" of risk-taking, directly seeking to depict (and condemn) authors Erik Rémès and Guillaume Dustan, the proselytizers of this religion.

Yet, what is this religion of risk-taking? We are obsessed with risk, which "has come to dominate individual and collective consciousness in the twenty-first century" (Denney 2005, 1). Hélène Joffe describes risk as "danger in modern clothes" (1999, 4). This manner of conceiving risk in terms of modernity allows for a connection with the notion of personal agency. That is, while humans have always been concerned with the ways in which things we value (such as health) are endangered, it was not until we moved beyond feudalism that we realized we had choice in the matter and that risk was tied to our decisions (Reith 2004, 386). The shift away from a destiny-focused view of risk has a significant impact on how we define risk. Once we accept that our future is the result of our decisions and not the master plan of an omnipotent being, risk is thus by definition *always* concerned with the future: what *will* happen to me as a result of my choices? This modern conception of risk has informed the reorganization of society in the name of mitigating risk rather than reacting to it: institutions, rules, laws, and technologies are formed for the purpose of communicating and regulating risk (Ericson and Haggerty 2001, 238). Political groups such as Act Up-Paris are one such example of an institution. While Act Up-Paris does advocate for the lives and health of

HIV-positive individuals (and, therefore, people whose risk of contamination has come to pass), their mission statement and their 1999 Pride public health campaigns are proof that Act Up-Paris is also concerned with the work of communication and regulation.

The large and evocative title of Act Up-Paris's campaign gives a name to the risky behavior that has formed the backbone of a "religion": fucking without a condom. In popular culture, this practice is known as barebacking. In the French context, Erik Rémès (directly named in the campaign) is perhaps one of the most well-known barebackers. In *Serial Fucker*, Rémès writes: "En France, le terme de bareback n'est pas encore très répandu. Seuls quelques initiés l'utilisent. Ce sont les mots qui créent les choses, les font naître. Sur les forums de discussion, peu à peu, le débat apparaît: Bareback pour ou contre? (2003)[2] [In France, the word bareback hasn't spread much. Only the initiated few use it. Words create things, give them life. The discussion is appearing, bit by bit, on discussion forums: bareback, for or against?][3] Here Rémès states that the act of naming the practice creates it. Whereas Rémès elsewhere describes barebacking as an "immediate sexuality" without barriers between partners, it is important to recognize that barebacking is indeed a creation (Rémès 2003, "Manifest du jus"). That is, while sex without condoms has always and will always exist, barebacking is a time-bound political statement against pro-condom advocates. As a creation of the barebackers, it comes with its own set of rules and expectations. These expectations are co-created by the members of the barebacking community, essentially establishing their own ethics of rawness.

Rawness spreads. Rémès reminds us that "depuis le milieu des années 90, le No Capote se popularise" ["Ever since the middle of the 90s, 'no condoms' has been getting popular"] citing the cases of HIV-positive porn stars who, shortly after infections reached their peak in 1994, abandoned condoms. Indeed, public health campaigns in France in the 1980s and 1990s largely took on the task of convincing the public to wear condoms. In the 1992 campaign by the Agence française de lutte contre le sida [French Agency Against AIDS][4], four young men in the *banlieue* are framed in medium closeup accompanied by the slogan "Les préservatifs: aujourd'hui tout le monde dit oui" ["Condoms. Today, everyone is saying yes"]. An alternate version also appeared, showing men in business suits. The framing of the photo and use of different types of models invites the (male) viewer to identify with the campaign. In so doing, it relies on the bandwagon mentality to convince the viewer to join "everyone" in saying yes to condoms. Other campaigns do not shy away from more sexualized portrayals in order to convince viewers that condoms can still be sexy/sensual: to name but two examples of campaigns, one might find a heterosexual couple making love and a muscular man's erect penis in a condom.

What ads such as these seek to do is promote a certain type of sexuality that is deemed responsible. By extension, anything that deviates from sex with condoms is then called irresponsible. All people are concerned with HIV, an axiom supported not only statistically but also by the breadth of individuals represented in public health campaigns. In this way, we are all living with AIDS, the disease being part of our societal fabric (Dean 1993, 84). It remains true, however, that gay men in particular bore much of the weight of the epidemic. The first mentions of HIV referred to it as a gay cancer. Early misconceptions of the disease linked HIV with gay men and sexual practices that popular culture dictates are commonplace in the community: sexual promiscuity, anal sex, and the use of poppers, for example (Perruchot 1981, 7). The promiscuity associated with gay men formed the base of the guilt gay men were subjected to, leading Bersani to a provisional conclusion that culpability is tied not only to "what" (anal sex between men) but also to how often (Bersani 1987, 210). In the same article, Bersani quotes outrageous claims made by medical professionals, depicting gay men flitting between 3000 men in a year (197). These public notions of HIV made policing gay men seem like a "moral imperative" (204). That is, the best way to control the disease was to control the men who were considered vessels of contagion. As such, "the sexual past was relentlessly reconfigured as a site of infectious irresponsibility" (Castiglia and Reed 2011, 3). Behaving irresponsibly was defined both in terms of having unprotected anal sex and in having it with a large number of partners. In response, gay men were asked either to adopt more normative sexual lifestyles or to abandon gay spaces that encouraged promiscuity such as bathhouses (Martel 1996, 326). Castiglia and Reed furthermore lament that the aforementioned reconfiguration represents a lost opportunity to celebrate the connections and support network that the past had created at a time when gay men needed it.

It is altogether unsurprising that shame was often the weapon of choice in advancing the pro-condom agenda. Consider again Act Up-Paris's 1999 campaign, the final lines of which recall the lost lovers and friends whose memory "spoils pleasure." Evoking what could only be described as survivor guilt is but one example of how "AIDS became a major shame-inflicting weapon" (Bersani and Phillips 2008, 31). There is a large corpus of scholarship on shame that shows the ways in which shame operates on our moral judgments which are in turn informed by what society sees as disgusting (see Menninghaus 2003; Miller 1997; Szabo 2009). For instance, Nussbaum reminds us that "societies ubiquitously select certain groups and individuals for shaming," going so far as to invent ways of branding those that they deem "abnormal" (2009, 174). What goes unspoken in her description is the power dynamic at play. One needs power in order to shame another person. Nussbaum goes on to describe the only individual who is above shame; he is, among other things, white, straight, and male (174). Outside of being a member of this narrow band of shameless persons, I argue that one can also avoid shame by rejecting the norms that govern it. By creating their own ethics of rawness, barebackers such as Erik Rémès and Guillaume Dustan allow us to see that terms like "responsibility" and "risk" do not have just one definition. Rémès writes, of Dustan, that "tout ce qu'il dit, c'est la libération de la honte d'être homo par la libération de la capote" ["Everything he says is the freedom from the shame of being gay via the freedom from the condom"] (Rémès 2003). Physically and ideologically speaking, barebacking is a path to freedom.

RESPONSIBILITY AND BUGCHASING

Rémès, sharing an account of a party at the Bareback House, a San Francisco club whose name reveals and revels in the debauchery that occurred within—that is, sex parties, which Michael Scarce describes as events where the receptive partner would service 20 insertive partners in a night (1999)—writes:

> Mars 1999. Fin de siècle. Samedi soir, Castro, le quartier gay de San Francisco. Direction la Bareback House. Le thème: "fuck the hole." Le droit d'entrée est de 8 dollars. Après avoir payé, Georges Butch, le boss, me tend le règlement intérieur: "ceci est une soirée bareback. Tous les invités sont présumés séropositifs ou alors ils ont pris la décision d'assister à ce genre de soirée. Par conséquent, il n'y aura pas de discussion sur le statut sérologique, la maladie ou la médecine. (Rémès 2003)
>
> March 1999. The turn of the century. Saturday Night, the Castro, the gayborhood of San Francisco. Heading to the Bareback House. The theme: "fuck the hole." Cover fee is 8 dollars. After having paid, Georges Butch, the boss, hands me the house rules: "this is a bareback party. All the guests are assumed to be HIV-positive or they have made the decision to attend this type of party. As a result, there will be no discussion about HIV status, the disease, or medicine.

In the above account, seropositivity is not a requirement for entry into this space, but the above quote demonstrates that seropositivity is an *assumption* within the walls of the Bareback House. Let us pretend for a moment that everyone at the Bareback House *is* HIV-positive (and not, as the host says, an HIV-negative individual who chose to attend anyway). In this context, our whole definition of risk *must* change. The need for a new definition of risk is why a pro-condom, anti-barebacking stance is ultimately ineffective in the context of the barebackers, even though it seems to be a logical extension of our concern with mitigating risk. Our concern with risk is aimed at *prevention, but that discourse falters when confronted with Rémès et al.'s ethics of* rawness. What, exactly, is the risk that Rémès is supposed to be mitigating? Considering that risk always belongs to the future and that Rémès is (already) HIV-positive, he has outlived his risk; infection is in his past and it can no longer be called risk at that point.

It is thus altogether fitting that Rémès quotes Butch's warning that there will be no talk about the disease, about HIV status, or the medicine used to treat it. Since naming something gives it life, it follows that not talking about risk is a way of denying its existence. In the absence of risk and the absence of discussing the disease, Rémès feels "Libre: descendu de la croix. À la Bareback House, je me sentais bien, sans complexe ni culpabilité (si un jour je l'ai jamais été . . .). Je me sentais libre. Délesté de toute honte. J'étais content et fier, heureux même. Ni mon homosexualité ni ma séropositivité n'étaient plus mon opprobre. [Free: let down from the cross. At the Bareback House, I felt good, no complexes, no guilt (as if I ever was guilty . . .). I felt free. Relieved from all shame. I was content and proud, happy even. Neither my homosexuality nor my HIV status was my burden to bear] (2003). Already, Rémès begins to show how barebackers reject the societal norms that would make them feel shame for engaging in certain behaviors. At the Bareback House, he feels no guilt, is relieved from shame, no longer feeling heteronormative society's reproach of his sexuality or his serological status.

This revelation is not necessarily groundbreaking. Over 20 years ago, Michael Scarce penned that "raw sex between positive men is often merely frowned upon, but when the partners are serodiscordant, words like murder and suicide enter the discussion" (1999). In the same article, Scarce adds that this is why an "HIVer" who is the insertive partner is seen as more guilty than the receptive partner. This point brings us to the other possible type of participant at the Bareback House: the HIV-negative participant who knowingly has chosen to attend the party. It is here that barebackers truly transgress our norms of responsibility: not only do HIV-positive individuals bear more of the blame, they are also asked to take on the onus of responsibility. Indeed, to join the festivities at the Bareback House, Rémès is asked to sign a waiver stating that he has no intention of contaminating anyone else, thus absolving the Bareback House of any liability. There is however no mention of a homologous form that an HIV-negative individual would have to sign, acknowledging the very real epidemiological risk to him.

The question that we must attempt to answer is whether having sex without a condom is an act of irresponsibility. For many individuals, I am sure it is considered irresponsible, yet it is important to conceive of irresponsibility not in terms of making a (bad) choice but rather in terms of being accountable for the choice that is made. That is to say that so long as one is aware of the risks or lack thereof, they are being responsible for their actions in a way that we may call being "accountable" and perhaps even "ethical." We also must consider the different ways that seropositive and seronegative individuals are asked to be held accountable for their actions. As demonstrated by Bersani and frequently lamented by Rémès in his corpus, seropositive individuals are asked to be more accountable for their actions and treated as killers if they fail to do so. For instance, we see in the 1990s the creation of disclosure laws in some countries such as the United States (where the Bareback House is located). These laws require that seropositive individuals share their status with sexual partners. Failing to do so could then result in punitive damages. Even in countries where it was not mandated by law, moral policing made it seem like the so-called responsible thing to do. This rationale is precisely why a venue such as the Bareback House asked its patrons to sign a declaration of honor that absolves the establishment from culpability should someone be infected with the virus. Porn stars such as Scott O'Hare, authors like Erik Rémès, and more widely barebackers as a group are making a choice to fight back against these discriminatory policies. O'Hare's declaration that he is no longer interested in ensuring that someone else remains negative could initially come off as being callous or selfish. It is much less a question of selfishness than it is an entreaty for all partners to *share* the responsibility, to be equally held accountable for their decisions.

Act Up-Paris's pointed references to Rémès and Dustan in their 1999 public health campaign is a sign of the type of moral policing that occurred around the barebackers. Even further, Rémès and Dustan are vilified for their actions. I wonder however if anyone at Act Up-Paris had *actually* taken the time to read their books. Seropositivity is omnipresent in both authors' corpuses and coexists with depictions of promiscuity, yet infection with HIV is not a requirement for existence in the worlds that Rémès and Dustan create. In fact, there are several instances in both novels where Rémès and Dustan discuss their decision to use condoms with their sexual partners or otherwise reveal that infecting their partners is *not* their objective. For Rémès, his decision is based on a desire for a more direct physical connection with his partners, one in which bodily fluids are freely exchanged. Even if he does not feel complete while wearing a condom he nevertheless notes: "Bien sûr, je peux faire avec. Je peux malgré tout bien bander et jouir" ["Of course, I can manage. I can, despite everything, get hard and come"] (Rémès 2003).

As far as Dustan is concerned, he describes a sexual experience with his lover Stéphane in which he has sex with condoms. A combination of the condoms and a poorly positioned sex sling makes it difficult for Dustan to reach orgasm. The two of them go home and Stéphane shares his desire to have sex without a condom. Still, Dustan resists the urge to ejaculate in his partner. This reluctance is despite Stéphane asking for it as he is sure that he is already seropositive. Dustan later discovers that Stéphane is in fact seronegative. Rather than being the monster that Act Up-Paris has made him out to be, Dustan makes a choice that protects his partner. Had Dustan actually penetrated his partner without a condom, we must still recognize that they would have followed the ethics of rawness that guide barebackers: Stéphane is aware of the danger, and in fact, assumes that his risk has already disappeared.

Stéphane's acceptance of his own risks lends itself to a discussion of another aspect of Rémès's definition of responsibility: being aware of the risks that one is taking. He turns to the Petit Larousse dictionary of the French language to define an irresponsible person as one who "n'est pas capable de répondre de ses actes, de sa conduite" ["is not responsible for his actions, for his behavior"] (2003). He goes on to clarify that gay people are quite informed, and for that reason, we cannot consider them to be irresponsible. The beauty, he says, of queerness is that gay men have always resisted having their sexuality delineated and the question of responsibility is no different for Rémès. As shown by Butch's proclamation upon entry in the Bareback House, gay men were well aware of any risk they may or may not be taking.

A skeptic reader may persist that barebackers were acting unfavorably in the middle of a pandemic, but a distinction must be made: risk mitigation must look different for barebackers because the risk itself is a different beast. Rémès writes that "je ne fais aucun prosélytisme du Bareback. Je pense plutôt faire de la prévention à ma manière" ["I'm not proselytizing for bareback sex in any way. Rather, I'm merely thinking of prevention in my own way"] (2003). Barebackers had different tools at their disposal, notably serosorting, whereby one sleeps only with men who have the same serostatus as oneself. We have already seen that risk is by its nature a forward-looking phenomenon. For gay men who have been infected with HIV, the risk of HIV infection disappears. Rémès describes how he came to be positive: "J'ai rencontré mon virus en 1989, quelques mois après mon arrivée à Paris. Vingt-quatre ans. Le coup de foudre. Prendre un premier X, aller à la gym, se faire un tattoo, devenir séropo, c'est le parcours classique du jeune pédé parisien normal" ["I met my virus in 1989, a few months after arriving in Paris. Twenty-four years old. Love at first sight. Taking X for the first time, going to the gym, getting a tattoo, getting AIDS, it's a normal young Parisian fag's classic path" (2003). At first glance, calling it a "parcours classique" [classic path] may lead one to believe that Rémès sees seroconversion as a predetermined destiny for gay men in Paris. However, he includes seroconversion in a list of other banal, everyday activities, much like it were a list of errands to run before the day is over. Each of these other activities are choices that one makes, choices for which Rémès is holding himself accountable. He continues to say that with the treatment methods available at the time, it was no longer a scary diagnosis (a sentiment echoed by Dustan as well, who compares HIV to a manageable disease such as diabetes) (2019, 85). The banalisation of the disease and indeed the lessening virulence of the disease certainly play a role in Act Up-Paris's anger toward Rémès and Dustan. In their campaign, they write that tritherapies, which put HIV-positive people "hors danger" [out of danger], invite everyone to enjoy sex without condoms. If there is no more danger to HIV-positive men, as Act Up-Paris admits, then it follows that there is also no more risk. This fact does not escape the barebackers. In their world, everyone is seropositive, or everyone assumes responsibility for participating in that world (Dustan 2019, 53). That world is inhabited by all sorts of people with various motivations. Rémès describes several different types of parties: all-positive parties, all-negative parties, Russian roulette parties (where seropositive and negative individuals are mixed without knowledge of one another's status) and conversion parties, events where men called bug chasers actively seek to become infected with HIV by positive men called gift givers.

In *Dans ma chambre* [*In My Room*], Dustan describes an episode in which he is playing the role of the insertive partner, which as we have seen, is frequently characterized as the more monstrous role. He writes:

> J'accélère pour qu'on en finisse. Quand il a joui je décule et j'enlève ma capote et je pense à lui gicler sur le trou et à étaler pour bien faire pénétrer la mort et je me branle et puis ma bite hyper tuméfiée reprend le dessus et comme je suis près de jouir je ne pense plus et puis j'explose en geyser et c'est comme dans un hyper bon film porno et tout de suite après je me remets à penser. (Dustan 2019, 62)
>
> [I speed up so that we can finish up. When he comes, I pull out and take off my condom and I think about coming on his hole and spreading it to penetrate him with death and I jerk off and then my swollen cock takes over and as I'm close to ejaculating I'm not thinking anymore and I explode like a geyser and it's just like in a really good porn film, and right away I start thinking again.]

Dustan's repeated use of the conjunction "and" is both remarkable and a raw style of writing that wraps the reader in what he is feeling in this moment. The polysyndeton seems to echo his own acceleration. It overwhelms and allows the reader to share, for a moment, the excitement that Dustan feels as he is reaching climax. For a brief moment, he fantasizes not simply about ejaculating on Stéphane, but on penetrating him with death. The "baiser de la mort" [the kiss of death], as both Rémès and Dustan refer to it, seems to carry with it a certain level of excitement and this excitement ultimately leads Dustan to orgasm. Once Dustan has achieved orgasm, he says that he begins to think again. If we recall the definition of responsibility as being accountable for one's acts, it seems here that Dustan, for a moment, is acting in an irresponsible way. He fantasizes about engaging in a destructive, raw act, and it is unclear what prevents him from doing so. It recalls, on the receptive side of the sex act, Bersani's vivid description of "women and gay men [who] spread their legs with an unquenchable appetite for destruction" (Bersani 1987, 211). We must distinguish, however, between a fantasy and the actual act of penetration. Blaming Dustan for being irresponsible is an unfair attribution of responsibility and goes against the ethics of rawness that govern barebacking. Responsibility is *shared*, and the partner Stéphane plays a role in the sexual act.

Furthermore, a compulsion toward or fetishization of destructive behavior cannot fully allow us to understand the phenomenon of bug chasing. Firstly, Bersani and Phillips remind us that the death drive alone is not sufficient to explain this phenomenon (Bersani and Phillips 2008, 35). Secondly, it unfairly vilifies sex partners as irresponsible. Earlier, I referred to a separate occasion in which Dustan had sex with Stéphane. In this other instance, Stéphane asks Dustan to have sex without a condom, saying that he feels he is already HIV-positive. Dustan refuses and later finds out that Stéphane was negative: "Je me dis que j'ai bien fait de ne pas jouir dans son cul. Et puis je me sens seul. Déçu. Et puis seul" ["I tell myself that I did well not to come in his ass. And then I feel alone. Disappointed. Then alone"] (Dustan 2019, 79). Dustan's sentences here are shorter. They are separated by punctuation, and the tone is sullen compared to the previous passage that I quoted. The two very different reactions to a similar situation demonstrate ways in which bug chasing might manifest itself. On one hand, there was excitement in taking a risk (or in Dustan's case, in *being* the risk). On the other hand, Dustan's disappointment and feeling of loneliness suggest an urge to feel connected to Stéphane. For the time being, Dustan inhabits a different, seropositive world than his lover. They are separated not only by condoms, but by the promise that Dustan will likely die and Stéphane will not.

In "Bareback Sex, Bug Chasers, and the Gift of Death," DeAnn K. Gauthier and Craig J. Forsyth identify four reasons that explain the phenomenon of bug chasing. Men seek contamination to be freed from fear of being infected, they eroticize risk-taking, they seek solidarity with their friends who have been infected, or they are taking political stands against stigmatization (1999, 93–95). Through the study of Dustan and Rémès, we can find evidence that supports these claims while gleaning a bit more understanding of the thought process behind bug chasing and gift giving.

> Si certains veulent tout partager, même leur Sida, c'est leur liberté. Tu piges? Qu'on soit pédé ou hétéro, la prévention est un acte perso que chacun doit intégrer, réfléchir et verbaliser. Il faut savoir quel est ton désir, sa force et ses

limites. En quoi la peur intervient sur ton désir? Jusqu'où tu veux prendre des risques? En quoi ce risque t'excite? C'est à toi de répondre. (Rémès 2003)

[If some people want to share everything, even their AIDS, that's their prerogative. Got it? Gay or straight, prevention is a personal act that everyone must integrate, reflect on, and put into words. You need to know your desire, its strength and its limits. When does fear intervene with your desire? How far will you go to take a risk? To what extent does this risk excite you? It's up to you to decide.]

Rémès uses the second person to interpelate the readers about their own desires, their own (pre)conceptions of barebacking, and what it means to be responsible. If, as we have seen, in the history of barebackers, the barebackers are often vilified for their irresponsibility, Rémès here turns it around and places the responsibility on the reader. The reader must determine what their own relationship with risk and excitement will be, and the reader must determine their own limits. It is not up to the barebacker alone to determine the limits, and the sharing of responsibility relieves the barebacker from the weight of all responsibility.

This position again differs from Act Up-Paris's campaign, which places the blame solely on the HIV-positive individual. The last line of their campaign reads that "le risque de contaminer ou d'être contaminé continue de gâcher notre plaisir" [the risk to infect or be infected continues to ruin our pleasure"]. It would then seem that the campaign places all responsibility on the HIV+ individual. Rémès rejects this assertion, preferring on many occasions to use the more active "se faire contaminer" ["to become infected"] suggesting that contamination is a personal choice for bug chasers, and that bug chasers are not *victims* but active participants in a decision to become contaminated. Bug chasers represent a unique subset of barebackers because they have successfully eroticized HIV and find appeal in HIV-infected semen (Scarce 1999). For Scarce, bug chasers carve out a tale of romance in which HIV is the ultimate connection that creates a "permanent partnership between lovers" (1999). Charged loads, as they come to be called, leave a permanent imprint on the recipient, unlike uninfected semen which disappears and leaves only the memory of an encounter. Bug chasers may see infection not as a death sentence but as the ultimate proof of love: "On peut se faire contaminer par amour. J'en connais de ces couples dont l'un était poz et l'autre neg. J'en ai vu des séroconversions amoureuses, des dons de son corps total, des virus en hostie. C'est toujours surprenant de voir deux personnes s'aimer au point de vouloir partager le virus de l'un d'eux" [One can get onself infected out of love. I know some of these couples where one is positive and the other negative. I've seen loving conversions, the gift of one's whole body, the virus as the body of Christ. It's always surprising to see two people who love each other to the point of wanting to share one of their viruses with the other] (Rémès 2003).

It is neither my prerogative nor my desire to determine which side is "right," but I do know that barebackers believed in their right to live their sexuality free from these stigmas. The ethics of rawness that they developed is why bareback parties came with their own set of assumptions. These assumptions are semantically empowering when compared to Act Up-Paris's campaign in which they speak of the fear of "being contaminated." Being contaminated insinuates passivity and victimhood. It strips the subject of its agency through the use of the passive voice. The barebackers are offering a chance to exercise agency not just to HIV-positive men but to HIV-negative ones as well. There can be no discussion of responsibility or irresponsibility because the assumption is that everyone made an informed decision, and it was a decision that they made themselves. These men may be accused of destroying themselves, but Rémès argues that they are instead fighting to build and defend their own identities: "Et bien non, nous ne sommes pas forcément autodestructeurs. Bien au contraire. Nous sommes en lutte pour nous assumer tels que nous sommes, tels que sont nos désirs. Vivre notre jouissance, respecter nos différences et agrandir notre liberté. Et notre liberté étend la vôtre à l'infini." [And no, we are not necessarily self-saboteurs. On the contrary. We are fighting to accept ourselves as we are, as we wish to be. To live our pleasure, to respect our differences, and to grow our freedom. And our freedom extends yours to infinity] (2003). This quote gets at the crux of the matter. Barebackers have felt the burden of responsibility placed on them by Act Up-Paris. They have felt pressure to behave in certain ways, but gay men "se sont toujours joués de la morale et des répressions" ["have always played with ethics and repression"] so that they could love according to their own rules (2003). Barebackers feel neither desire nor obligation to allow Act Up-Paris to repress their sexuality through morality no more than they feel that gay men as a whole community should conform to heteronormative ideas of what love should look like. Barebackers engaged in an ethics of rawness that allowed them to act in their own interest, but, in their own way, they act in the interests of all gay men, HIV-positive and HIV-negative alike.

CONTEMPORARY REPRESENTATIONS OF RISK

We are now more than two decades removed from the height of HIV infections. Furthermore, the use of medication to *prevent* HIV infection rather than treat it is becoming more popular. Our evolving conceptions of HIV risk have resulted in cultural productions that respond to this shift. Analysis of a 2018 public health campaign alongside *Théo et Hugo dans le même bateau* shows how our contemporary perceptions of risk have influenced cultural productions. Earlier, I staked the claim that barebacking is a time-bound phenomenon, placing it squarely in the mid-1990s as a political statement. Does this definition mean that barebacking is dead? The answer is complex. In terms of the definition that I have given it, then yes, barebacking does not exist anymore. Popular parlance would disagree, as the term bareback has been reappropriated in the 21st century to refer to sex without condoms. For my purposes, I refer to sex without condoms as precisely that: condomless sex. It is not barebacking because it does not respond to the same political climate, it does not belong to the same *ethics* of rawness (if it ever could). Nor is it, I will argue, unprotected sex, because our definition of protection has expanded.

The current stakes of the virus can in large part be reduced to two simple acronyms: U=U and PrEP (and to a lesser extent PEP). U=U stands for Undetectable = Untransmittable (in French, *indétectable* = *intransmissible*). It has been discovered that if an HIV-positive individual's viral load drops low enough that it is no longer detectable, that person cannot transmit the disease. While treatment has, for many years, placed seropositive individuals out of danger as Act Up-Paris has worded it, the U=U revelation also alleviates the possibility that the HIV-positive individual can pose any danger to seronegative individuals. Immediately, we see how traditional views of barebacking and bug chasing begin to break down, unable to stand the test of time and the improvement of medicine. If U=U is a boon for HIV-positive people, PrEP and PEP directly implicate HIV-negative individuals. PrEP and PEP stand for, respectively, pre-exposure prophylaxis and post-exposure prophylaxis. In the case of PrEP, HIV-negative men begin a regimen of medication (a combination of drugs such as Truvada or Descovy) that prevents HIV infection. There are two main dosing recommendations: one pill daily, or an on-demand format that consists of a two-pill booster before a sexual rapport followed by two one-pill doses 24 and 48 hours after sex. PEP, as the name indicates, is used when someone suspects that they may have been exposed to the virus. It is an intensive daily regimen of medication that attacks the virus before it can take hold of the body.

The public health campaigns that I have looked at thus far have considered the use of condoms as the most logical response to the HIV/AIDS crisis. Indeed, faced with the possibility of infection, our first reaction is often to create a border in order to stop the flow of traffic. One need not look very hard for examples of this reaction, particularly in recent memory. When a deadly coronavirus appeared in a Wuhan market in December 2019, the world responded by mandating face masks and closing borders. Even within the Schengen zone, Europeans were restricted, unable to move between countries in order to contain a virus that quickly spread across the globe. Yet U=U, PrEP, and PEP perturb our very understanding of what it means to stop the spread of a disease. In the history of AIDS, there has always been a mistrust of bodily fluids. The containment of those fluids is a logical response. Science, however, no longer supports condoms (and condoms alone). In the United States, the CDC (Centers for Disease Control) hosts an online HIV risk reduction tool. The user begins by providing information concerning what was done (anal sex, oral sex), who did it (serostatus), and how the partners were protected (condoms, PrEP for an HIV-negative partner, or TasP [treatment as prevention] for an HIV-positive partner). The tool then provides the chance that HIV infection occurs. The results might be shocking: anal sex with a condom is in fact *more likely* to result in infection than anal sex on PrEP (no condom). Suddenly, we find that our definition of risk has changed, causing with it a shift in risk mitigation, perceptions of risk, and cultural productions of risk itself.

In 2018, AIDES, another HIV advocacy group in France, produced a series of three public health posters that were distributed around the country. The purpose of this campaign was to spread information about PrEP, still rather new in this country at that time. The three versions of the campaign can be consulted on their website under the campaign's official title, Prep 4 Love. All three versions are structured similarly: they feature black-and-white images of couples locked in an intimate embrace that intertwines their bodies. The poses suggest a lack of separation between lovers, already hinting at the new types of discourse we are poised to have thanks to PrEP. The different versions of the poster attempt to speak to the different demographics of people who might lay eyes upon it: a heterosexual white couple, a biracial male homosexual couple, and a heterosexual couple of African descent. Unlike earlier examples of public health campaigns which stressed the importance of condoms or tried to convince the viewer that sex could be enjoyable *despite* condoms, they are completely absent from the 2018 campaign. Catchphrases, scrawled in white over the skin of the models, suggest a very different approach to sex in a world where PrEP is available. The viewer is told to "propagate heat," "catch desire," and "spread passion." These verbs recall the language typically associated with disease and epidemics. Here they are reappropriated and stripped of their virulent nature, instead being used to share positive things associated with sex and love. Anything except the virus. A simple slogan is common to all three versions of the poster: "un comprimé par jour vous protège du VIH" ["one pill a day protects you against HIV"]. Paired with the models, all of whom are conventionally attractive, happy, and who are presented as healthy individuals, this campaign promotes the message that sex and good health can exist together. Unlike previous models that advocated for condom use, this campaign reestablishes the possibility of an unhindered connection between partners. Baudrillard reminds us that in a modern society, "le sexe, l'argent, l'information doivent circuler librement" ["sex, money, information must circulate freely"] (Baudrillard 1990, 72). Revoking sexuality to curb the risk of viral transmission, for Baudrillard, is absurd.

The arrival of PrEP as a tool of prevention will also have longterm effects on what it means to be *responsible* in an epidemic. Rather, it will change *who* will be responsible. As noted by David Caron in "Truvada mon amour," the traditional model places all the responsibility on the HIV-positive individual to disclose his status. Faithfully respecting a PrEP regimen eliminates the risk of seroconversion, thus rendering obsolete the need to know the partner's status. Additionally, it is the responsibility of the HIV-negative person to follow their own regimen: "PrEP revives the idea of shared responsibility for the burden of HIV infection" (2014). This dynamic is another reason why it is difficult (or impossible) to think of barebacking in today's world. There is, rather, a new way for men to have sex without condoms, "as nature intended" (Ibid.). In 2017, François Berdougo and Gabriel Girard published their book *La fin du sida est-elle possible?* [*Is the End of AIDS Near?*] and lament that while there is a great need to remember the past that has led us to our present moment, contemporary narratives have a hard time making their voices known (161). Caron sees this as an attempt to anchor our history in the grander scheme of American (or Western) history. I have argued elsewhere, though, that we see the HIV/AIDS epidemic as a cultural trauma and as such, it continues to resurface until such time that we can put the ghosts of that past to rest (Troth 2021). We are not there yet. In the United States, PrEP can be cost-prohibitive; talking about sex and particularly anal sex (between men) is still a taboo subject. Merely evoking it gets more attention than the medication that public health campaigns are attempting to promote. We do, however, see at least one cultural production that subscribes to this new narrative. Ducastel and Martineau's 2016 film *Théo et Hugo dans le même bateau* [*Paris 5:59: Theo and Hugo*] tells the story of a condomless encounter in a sex club between Théo, an HIV-negative man, and Hugo, who is both HIV-positive and undetectable. There are traces of the old, culpabilizing narrative present in *Théo et Hugo*. Théo cries because he feels stupid for having taken a risk. Hugo scolds him for not knowing better while going to a sex club. There is an old man in a hospital waiting room that calls them homophobic slurs. Despite these examples, there are glimpses into a much brighter future. Théo did not ask Hugo what his status was before they had sex; Hugo did not feel pressured to disclose his status in the heat of the moment. Because Hugo's viral load is undetectable, he never really posed any threat to Théo. Finally, because Théo begins a post-exposure treatment, he accepts that he be held accountable for his actions. By Rémès's definition of what it means to be responsible, we would certainly find it difficult to call either character "irresponsible."

Even though I distinguish barebacking from having condomless sex, there are some connections that become clear thanks to the ethics of rawness that came from the barebackers. Responsibility is shared among partners, and when risk becomes so small that it is nearly negligible, gay men respond appropriately. They adjust their behaviors based on what they believe the risk to be. Rémès, as it turns out, was right in saying that the barebackers' freedom would extend *everyone's* freedom. Dustan passed away in 2005. Rémès is still alive. In 2017, he published a collection of his own work. In it, a particularly-relevant passage appears: "De nos jours, un maximum de gays baisent sans capotes. C'est un fait statistique. Même et surtout les jeunes. Qu'on la veuille ou non, Dustan et moi avions raison: la capote est insupportable à terme" ["Nowadays, most gays are fucking without condoms. It's a statistical fact. Even and especially the young ones. Whether you want it or not, Dustan and I were right: condoms are insufferable after a while] (Rémès 2017, 14). It seems that Dustan and Rémès were somewhat clairvoyant in their estimation of the future of the HIV/AIDS epidemic. We cannot say that there is *no* risk, but what we can say is that the risk has changed and is sometimes so small that it becomes negligible. Natural sex, or sex without condoms, can exist between men with little fear of viral repercussions. Responsibility does not look the same today as it did in the 1980s or 1990s, nor should it. Of course, natural sex between men will always be seen as *unnatural* by some in the heteronormative world, yet that is the beauty of queerness that Rémès and Dustan have revealed through writing: sometimes we have much to lose from accepting heteronormative definitions of sexuality and everything to gain by rejecting them.

BIBLIOGRAPHY

Baudrillard, Jean. 1990. "Prophylaxie et Virulence." La Transparence du mal. Paris: Éditions Galilée.

Berdougo, François and Gabriel Girard. 2017. *La fin du sida est-elle possible?* Paris: Editions Textuel, 2017.

Bersani, Leo. 1987. "Is the Rectum a Grave?" *AIDS: Cultural Analysis/Cultural Activism*. Vol. 43.

Bersani, Leo and Adam Phillips. 2008. "Shame on You." *Intimacies*. Chicago: University of Chicago Press.

Caron, David. 2014. "Truvada mon amour." Brooklyn Quarterly.

Castiglia, Christopher and Christopher Reed. 2011. "Introduction: In the Interest of Time." In *If Memory Serves: Gay Men, AIDS, and the Promise of the Queer Past*. Minnesota Scholarship Online, https://minnesota.universitypressscholarship.com/view/10.5749/minnesota/9780816676101.001.0001/upso-9780816676101-chapter-1.

Cheng, Jih-Fei, et al. 2020. "Introduction." In *AIDS and the Distribution of Crises*, edited by Jih-Fei Cheng, et al., Durham: Duke University Press, 1–28.
Dean, Tim. 1993. "The Psychoanalysis of AIDS." October, Vol. 63 (Winter), 83–116.
Denney, David. 2005. *Risk and Society*. London: Sage Publications, 2005.
Ducastel, Olivier and Jacques Martineau (dir.). 2016. *Théo et Hugo dans le même bateau*: France, 97 min.
Dustan, Guillaume. [1996] 2019. *Dans ma chambre*. Paris: P. O. L.
Ericson, Richard V. and Kevin D. Haggerty. 2001. "The Police of Risk." In T. Baker and J. Simon eds. *Embracing Risk*. Chicago: Chicago University Press, 2001, 238–72.
Gauthier, DeAnn K. and Craig J. Forsyth. 1999. "Bareback Sex, Bug Chasers, and the Gift of Death." *Deviant Behavior: An Interdisciplinary Journal*, 20: 85–100.
Joffe, Hélène. 1999. *Risk and the "Other."* Cambridge: Cambridge University Press.
Menninghaus, Winfried. 2003. *Disgust: Theory and History of a Strong Sensation*. Trans. by Howard Eiland and Joel Golb. Albany: State University of New York Press.
Miller, William Ian. 1997. *The Anatomy of Disgust*. Cambridge, MA: Harvard University Press:
Nussbaum, Martha C. 2009. "Inscribing the Face: Shame and Stigma." In *Hiding from Humanity*. Princeton, NJ: Princeton University Press.
Reith, Gerda. 2004. "Uncertain Times: The Notion of 'Risk' and the Development of Modernity." In *Time and Society*. London: Sage Publications.
Rémès, Erik. 2003. *Serial Fucker*. Paris: Editions Blanche. Amazon Kindle eBook.
———. *Pride*. 2017. Montreuil-Bellay: Musardine.
Scarce, Michael. 1999. "A Ride on the Wild Side." *Poz*. https://www.poz.com/article/A-Ride-on-the-Wild-Side-1460-8374Snorton, C. Riley. "Afterword." AIDS and the Distribution of Crises, edited by Jih-Fei Cheng, et al., Duke University Press, 2020, pp. 313–317.
Szabo, Jason. 2009. "Death, Decay, and the Genesis of Shame." In *Incurable and Intolerable: Chronic Disease and Slow Death in Nineteenth-Century France*. New Brunswick, NJ: Rutgers University Press.
Troth, Brian. 2021. "Haunted Spaces: Trauma, Mourning, and Melancholia in the HIV Epidemic in France." *Contemporary French Civilization*, 42, 2, 129–46.

NOTES

1. They can be consulted online by name of the campaign through the University of Rochester's AIDS Education Collection. The archives are located at https://digitalcollections.lib.rochester.edu/.
2. I have used a Kindle eReader version of *Serial Fucker*.
3. All translations are my own, unless noted otherwise.
4. This campaign image can be consulted at https://collections.nlm.nih.gov/catalog/nlm:nlmuid-101450075-img.

Chapter Five

"C'est Votre Choix" or, Private Identities and Public Militancy in the Second Decade of the AIDS Epidemic in France

The Case of Gay Porn Magazine Projet X

João Florêncio

HOMOSEXUALITY AND AIDS BEYOND US HEGEMONY

The writing of gay histories has tended to privilege as its actors both activists involved in the fight for gay liberation and, later, LGBTQ+ rights. Often centered in organizations such as the Wissenschaftlich-humanitäres Komitee (Scientific-Humanitarian Committee) in Germany, the Cultuur en Ontspanningscentrum (Center for Culture and Leisure) in the Netherlands, the Mattachine Society and the Gay Liberation Front (GLF) in the United States, Arcadie and the FHAR or Front Homosexuel d'Action Révolutionnaire (Homosexual Front for Revolutionary Action) in France, or the Homosexual Law Reform Society, Gay Left and OutRage! in the UK, those histories have often painted a picture of a gay community brought together by shared political ambitions hovering between a revolutionary ethos of liberation and a liberal realpolitik of equality as the post-war decades went by. In the context of such tension between Left-revolutionary narratives of liberation and neoliberal understandings of equality, different scholars have favored rather diverse, albeit not mutually exclusive, entry points into the histories of the homosexuality. Some, like David K. Johnson (2019), have highlighted the role of capitalist consumer cultures in the formation of a sense of community among gay men. Others, like Aaron Lecklider (2021), chose instead to focus on the influence of leftist ideologies and political organizing on what would eventually become the gay movement.

The writing of gay histories of AIDS in the Global North has tended to follow a similar path, one that has centered on histories of activism. That connection between homosexual and AIDS activism has perhaps been most famously articulated by Douglas Crimp, who, in 1987—six years after the first cases of what would come to be known as AIDS were first noted in the United States—argued for the indebtedness of early gay AIDS organizations like the Gay Men's Health Crisis (GMHC) to the political history of the gay activism. In his words:

> Though it may be true that few, if any, of the founders of the GMHC were centrally involved in gay politics, everything they were able to accomplish—from fundraising and recruiting volunteers to consulting with openly gay health care professionals and getting educations out to the gay community—depended on what had already been achieved by the gay movement. (1987, 250)

For Crimp, writing against other activists like Larry Kramer or writer Randy Shilts, the accomplishments of gay AIDS organizations had been possible because gay men had already come together as a community through an earlier collective embrace of sex and of sexual politics. It was our "conscious work on our own sexualities that [had] allowed many of us to change our sexual behaviors" and take on safer sex (253). Because gay men were already so open and experimental with regards to sexuality and promiscuity, the introduction of safer-sex measures like condom use could be incorporated within the ethics of sexual experimentation, openness and liberation that were already established when AIDS first hit our public consciousness. Condoms and therefore safer sex, Crimp argues, were a way not only to save lives but also to ensure the survival of the politics of promiscuity around which gay men had rallied a decade before. It was for that reason that, to him, "all productive practices concerning AIDS [would] remain at the grassroots level" (265).

Gay histories of AIDS have thus projected an image of activist organizations campaigning and demonstrating against the slow response of governments and pharmaceutical companies and working on the ground to hand out information and condoms in the community, following a principle whereby better information would necessarily result in informed safer-sex choices

(Warner [1995] 2009; Schulman 2021). According to these narratives, the 1980s saw a political re-awakening among gay men who, faced with the tragedy of AIDS and the slow responses of governments and the pharmaceutical industry, came together to demand support and research, all while often trying to rid themselves of the image of promiscuous irresponsibility and arrested development with which they had become associated as a result of the sexual revolution and its 1970s gay liberation aftermath (Halkitis 2000; Shepard 2001; Richardson 2005; Schulman 2012; Andersson 2018). Contemporary media narratives of the period such as David France's documentary *How to Survive a Plague* (2012) or Robin Campillo's drama *120 BPM* (2017), too, privilege activist actors in their AIDS narratives, favoring grassroots campaigning as *the* history that ought to be remembered. In so doing, they represent a form of AIDS media "retroactivism" that draws from and remakes AIDS cultural and political imaginaries to reimagine and reinvigorate contemporary struggles and forms of community organizing (Hilderbrand 2006; Ledin 2021).

Activism is only one of many aspects of gay histories and of gay men's response to AIDS, however. The broader picture is messier than that. Not only have AIDS activists had a series of infamous split-ups and heated disagreements on tactics and strategy very much since the beginning of the crisis, but the image of sexual responsibility and safer-sex compliance that has come to be associated with gay AIDS activists fails to capture the ethical dilemmas and complexities of everyday gay lives and sexual cultures. As Sarah Schulman notes in her recent history of ACT UP New York, "for the first few years of ACT UP safe sex was de rigueur, but then it started to break down, in part from AIDS exhaustion" (2021, 352). As a result, tensions started unfolding between the activist spokespersons for the "community" and those gay men who—for whatever reasons—were not living their lives according to the principles and image of sexual responsibility the activist organizations were trading for effective political lobbying and to incentivize allyship among the wider population. In the words of Michael Warner, reflecting on his own condomless sex encounters in the early 1990s:

> The appeal of queer sex, for many, lies in its ability to violate the responsibilizing frames of good, right-thinking people. AIDS education, in contrast, often calls for people to affirm life and see sex as a healthy expression of self-esteem and respect for others . . . Most efforts to encourage us to take care of ourselves through safer sex also invite us to pretend that our only desire is to be proper and good. ([1995] 2009, 165)

Notwithstanding the damage that centering histories of AIDS in the Global North has done to how HIV is perceived, lived, and dealt with in the Global

South—in the highly gendered and racialized contexts of global capitalism and the ongoing legacies of colonialism (Cheng, Juhasz, and Shahani 2020)—the dominant narratives of gay AIDS activism in the Global North itself also fail to sufficiently account for national differences and the particularities of local histories. The historical narratives that privilege gay AIDS activists owe part of their longevity to the global hegemony of the United States in the cultural and political outputs of the AIDS crisis. Indeed, just by looking at histories of AIDS and AIDS activism in Europe, one comes to realize the degree to which the model of AIDS activism that has become cemented in our consciousness as a defining part of late 20th-century gay histories is insufficient when trying to grapple with histories of HIV and AIDS outside the United States. It would suffice to look at countries like Germany or Portugal to realize that histories of AIDS that center gay activists organized against political institutions cannot account for how the crisis unfolded in those European nations, whether in terms of how activists organized, how they related to the state, or the role of AIDS itself in shaping the identity of a pre-existing gay political constituency in the later decades of the 20th century. As António Fernando Cascais notes with regards to the history of societal responses to AIDS in Portugal, these took precisely the opposite form of their US equivalent. While, in the United States, a pre-existing gay community already politically organized was able to respond to the social backlash against gay men triggered by AIDS, in Portugal—a country that lived under dictatorship between 1926 and 1974—it was the fight against AIDS that created, for the first time, a visible Portuguese gay political constituency (Cascais 2006). If, as Crimp had claimed, it was the pre-existing grassroots gay movement that would be responsible for "all productive practices concerning AIDS," the reality in Portugal could not have been more different. While some gay men became deeply involved in the Portuguese organizations that emerged in response to AIDS, those organizations had been created and led by health professionals and a few public figures driven by principles of the "common good," human rights, and citizenship. They were not, in sum, grassroots organizations—let alone grassroots *gay* organizations—like those that appeared in the United States and which have become privileged actors in the contemporary AIDS imaginary. As a result, the fact that the fight against AIDS in Portugal was born uncoupled from gay activism led the cause to have a much higher level of public acceptance than it had been the case in the United States (Cascais 2006).

Germany, too, offers an alternative history of AIDS activism, one that differs both from the hegemonic US model and from that of Portugal. There, the Deutsche AIDS-Hilfe (German AIDS-Relief) was created in 1985 as a national umbrella organization that brought together different gay-led regional organizations that had emerged independently throughout West Germany. Its formation was indeed facilitated by the Federal Centre for Health Education and it would come to be funded by the federal government on the basis that it would serve as mediator between the state and its homosexual citizens (Freeman 1992; Haus 2016). The Deutsche AIDS-Hilfe and its relationship to the state therefore embody a history of AIDS activism that is rather different from that of the United States, where in 1987 Republican Senator for North Carolina Jesse Helms famously introduced an amendment to a Labor, Health and Human Services bill which sought to prevent public funds to be allocated to sexual health campaigns seen to promote or condone homosexual acts (Crimp 1987; Meyer 2003). Or, for that matter, different too from that of the UK, where the conservative government of Margaret Thatcher introduced Section 2a to the Local Government Act 1988 (commonly known as Section 28), which prohibited local authorities from "promoting" homosexuality in schools as a result of an increase in stigmatization of homosexuals due to the AIDS crisis.

Hegemonic historical narratives of AIDS activism are therefore insufficient to capture not only the complexities and even contradictions of gay lives and sex cultures during the first decades of the epidemic, but also the specificities of how AIDS, its cultures, and activism have been lived in different national contexts. For the remainder of this article I will focus on a particular case study drawn from the French context, namely, how HIV, AIDS, and safer-sex messaging were featured alongside raw depictions of and references to sexual behaviors deemed "risky" in hardcore gay porn magazine *Projet X* (1995–2000). In so doing, my aim is to map the ways in which notions of safety and risk, private and public, autonomy and consent, played out and were negotiated on the pages of the magazine. From there, I will discuss them in relation to the particular ways in which discourses and politics of identity and citizenship unfolded in the context of the Fifth Republic. Focusing on the rawness of how *Project X* navigated the political landscape of sexual risk, pleasure, and autonomy during the second decade of the AIDS epidemic will offer an important subcultural contribution to the broadening of AIDS histories and cultures during the first two decades of the epidemic. It will allow me to foreground the dialectical tensions between both universalism and communitarianism, and private and public at the heart of French national identity and how those have shaped the specificities of gay men's engagement with AIDS—or lack thereof—at the dawn of the 21st century.

PROJET X: THE RAW AND THE COOKED

Launched in November of 1994 by publisher Joël Hladynink and editor Olivier Planque, the inaugural series of *Projet X* included only three issues before it folded in January 1995 "due to a number of problems" (*Projet X*

31, 31). Relaunched in November 1995 under the new editorship of François Agrapart ("Dick," his *nom de plume*), the second series of the magazine ran for 50 issues until April 2000, changing editor once along the way, from issue 32 (July 1998) onward. Directed at a readership that was "gay, kinky, hard and into forms of sex that are marginal, if not completely weird" (*Projet X* 31, 31), the magazine offered some gay men a platform to explore, discuss, fantasize, and learn about forms of sexuality that went well beyond penile penetration. Those included, among other practices: bondage, sadomasochism, domination and submission, fisting, piercing, urophagia and coprophagia, exhibitionism and public sex, fetishes such as leather, sports kit, trainers, military or punk looks, rape fantasies, and—central to my argument—raw eroticizations of ejaculate at a time when condom use was very much the single strategy to tackle the epidemic. Like all other gay porn magazines published during the 1990s, *Projet X* had to find ways to balance the no-limits sexual adventurousness expected by its readers with a civic responsibility to offer information on safer-sex practices. Already issue 2 of the second series (December 1995) included an infographic on safer sex which, according to the editorial, would be "to the taste" of the readership (1). Taking into account the sexual practices of its target market, the magazine published for the first time in that number an illustrated guide on reducing the risk of HIV transmission by using gloves during fisting, washing sex toys, using condoms when fucking, consuming one's own feces rather than someone else's, and covering any wounds resulting from S&M play with bandages.

At the same time, however, a disclaimer published, with virtually the same wording, in every issue of the magazine hinted at a more nuanced approach to sexual risk-taking.

> Le contenu de ce magazine peut être choquant du fait des pratiques sexuelles décrites et mise en scène. Nous vous conseillons donc de ne mettre cette revue qu'entre les mains de personnes au fait de nos pratiques ou dûment mise en garde!
>
> Notre position est que tout se résout dans le libre consentement, en tout conscience de son partenaire. Nous vous recommandons d'appliquer les règles du sexe sans risque (préservatif, nettoyage du matos, gants . . .). Cette revue ne doit en aucun cas être mise entre les mains de mineurs. (*Projet X* 15, 1)
>
> [The content of this magazine may be shocking due to the sexual practices described and represented. We therefore advice that you only put this magazine in the hands of people who familiar with our practices or who have been duly warned.
>
> Our position is that everything gets figured out through the free and conscious consent of your partner. We recommend that safe sex rules are followed

(condoms, cleaning of toys, gloves . . .). This magazine must never be put in the hands of minors].

The magazine's safer-sex recommendations were concomitant with an editorial line that refused to police content seen to carry out greater risks of HIV transmission, as alluded to by the above disclaimer and further evidenced by the editorial published in the very same issue of January 1997:

> J'ai entendu ici ou là à propos de Projet X quelque chose qui portrait se résumer de façon lapidaire par "Toujours plus?" Notre réponse: "Certainement pas!"
>
> Notre but n'est pas, à l'instar de l'émission la plus racoleuse du PAF (paysage audiovisuel français), de vous prouver que tout est possible! Projet X, de par son mode de distribution, ne se veut ni exhibitionniste ni prosélyte. Nous ne souhaitons pas surfer sur la vague du hard comme cela se fait dans la presse plus ou moins grand public. Notre objet est bien au contraire de partager avec un public averti les connaissances que nous avons et que nous récoltons au fil des rencontres. Ce partage des connaissances a pour but:
>
> - de s'épanouir en leur montrant qu'ils ne sont pas seuls et que toutes les formes de sexualité qui ne mettent pas en cause le consentement de leur partenaire et le cadre légal sont respectables,
> - d'indiquer à tous les dangers potentiels des pratiques les plus hard,
> - d'aider autant que faire se peut les associations et les différents acteurs de la scène hard.
>
> En matière de prévention, nous vous conseillons bien entendu des pratiques sans risques. Cependant, certains d'entre vous ont des rapports non protégés: c'est votre choix. Nous pensons qu'il ne nous appartient pas de les censurer. Ceci reviendrait simplement à occulter le problème, à le déplacer hors de la vue de tous en un endroit où personne ne cherchera jamais à lui apporter de solution. (1)
>
> [I've heard something here and there about Project X that could be summed up succinctly as "Always more?" Our answer: "Certainly not!"
>
> Our goal is not to prove to you that everything is possible, like the most racy show in the French audiovisual landscape! Project X, by its mode of distribution, is neither exhibitionist nor proselytizing. We do not wish to surf on the wave of hardcore as it is done in the press more or less aimed at the general public. On the contrary, our aim is to share with an informed public the knowledge that we have and that we gather through our sexual encounters. This sharing of knowledge is intended to:

- to help some people to blossom by showing them that they are not alone and that all forms of sexuality that do not call into question legal frameworks and the consent of their partner are respectable,
- to point out to all the potential dangers of the most hardcore practices,
- to help as much as possible the associations and the different actors of the hard scene.

As far as prevention is concerned, we of course advise you to adopt safer-sex practices. However, some of you have unprotected sex: it's your choice. We do not think it is appropriate to censure it. To do so would simply be to hide the problem, to move it out of sight to a place where no one will ever try to solve it.]

It was likely due to this approach that sought to provide safer-sex information while simultaneously refusing to censor content that flew in the face of a safer-sex consensus always more idealized than actual that *Projet X* regularly published personal classified ads by men seeking "no-taboo" condomless sex, ads that were therefore especially raw when compared to the ones circulating around the same time in anglophone gay publications. Ads of this kind were included in every single issue of the magazine's 5-year run, starting before the implementation of highly active antiretroviral therapies (HAART) as successful drug regimens for the management of HIV infection and continuing even while HAART had not yet been found to also prevent viral transmission. For instance, in issue 2 (December 1995), the following ad appeared written in both French and English, two pages after the safer-sex infographic mentioned earlier:

ANIMAL SEX

Mec 33a. 1m73 68 kg, pas mal foutu, plombé mais pas dépressif cherche mecs pour vidanges en tous genres. Belle queue active et pisseuse. Bouche baveuse, pompeuse et bouffeuse de culs. Ouvert à toutes propositions dégueulasses de mecs vicelards et très pervers mais cools. Rasés, tatoués, percés, avec cul et queue juteux. Bouffage et toutes pratiques réciproques. Gang-Bang.

ANIMAL SEX

Man 33yrs., 1m73, 68kg, O.K. body, HIV+ but not depressed seeks guys wanting to empty themselves. Good juicy active pissing cock, watering mouth for arse fucking and licking out. All filthy suggestions considered from vicious, perverse yet easy-going, shaved, pierced, tattooed guys with juicy cocks. All activities reciprocal. Gang-bang. (*Projet X* 2, 57)

Three numbers later, in issue 5 (March 1996), and this time only in French, another advertiser stated his pursuits so clearly it becomes even harder to reconcile them with the axiomatic logics of "SSR" or "*sex sans risque*" (safe sex) that had become hegemonic in mainstream gay public discourse during the 1980s and '90s:

> VIDANGEUR DE FOUTRE
>
> Belle gueule de salope 29a., 1m74, 70 kg, tifs courts, teube 19 cm, cul et couilles rasés. Bon tire-jus pour males actifs BM/TBM, remplisseurs et gaveurs de foutre. Plans directs avec mecs qui veulent se vidanger dans cul et gueule endurants. Tous plans, partouzes, abattage, chantier, foyer. Adore godes, cire, fist, uro, bondage, pinces. (61–62)
>
> [DRAINER OF SPUNK
>
> Beautiful slut mouth 29, short hair, cock 19cm, shaved ass and balls. Good juice-drainer for WE/VWE active men, fillers and cum feeders. Straightforward scenes with blokes who want to empty themselves inside a strong ass and mouth. All scenes, orgies, humiliation, building sites, home. Love dildos, wax, fist, piss, bondage, clamps.]

When compared to equivalent magazines published elsewhere such as US-based *Drummer*, which had been launched in 1975, *Projet X* stands out by the rawness with which it refuses to either censure or censor from its pages references to sexual activities more likely to increase the risk of HIV transmission. Furthermore, and unlike *Drummer*, which had seen an increase in editorial pieces about AIDS, AIDS activism, and safer sex, as well as a drastic reduction in references to eroticized bodily fluids in its classifieds section as the 1980s and 1990s unfolded (Florêncio 2020, 43), *Projet X*'s only editorial reference to safer sex was the safer-sex infographic that appeared in every single issue of the magazine from December 1995 onward, often near personal classifieds such as the one below, published in French, English, and German in issue 33 (1998):

> RÉSERVOIR À FOUTRE—PARIS
>
> 35a., 1m85, 78 kg, brun, imberbe, musclé, percé, offre beau fion à doser et tasser, no capote, uro, gode, fist, abattage, partouze, exhib. Cherche mec ou groupe de mecs, gros juteurs, aimant vraie salope à gaver cul et gueule. Inversion des rôles possible, réponse assure, déplacement sur l'Europe, peux recevoir.
>
> CUM RESERVOIR—PARIS
>
> 35 years, 1m85, 78kg, brown hair, shaven, muscley, pierced, offers beautiful hole to cram and fill, no condoms, uro, dildo, fist, group sex, orgy, exhibition. Looking for guy or group of guys, who cum a lot, who like stuffing a real whore's arse and mouth. Possible to switch roles, reply guaranteed, voyages throughout Europe, can accommodate.

D SPERMATANK—PARIS

> 35/185/78, braun, unbehaart, muskulös, gepierct, bietet sein Arschloch zum Abfüllen und Vollpumpen, ohne Gummi, mit Pisse, Dildo, Fist, Gruppenfick, Outdoor, zeigegeil. Suche Kerl oder Gruppe, fette Abspritzer, die eine echte Schlampe zum Abfüllen von Fresse und Arsch mögen. Rollentausch möglich, Antwort garantiert, reise in Europa, kann beherbergen. (76)

As pornographic illustrations, comic strips, and written porn fictions involving condomless sex were also common in magazines like *Drummer* throughout the AIDS crisis, *Projet X* does stand out not because it included pornographic fantasies that many would not feel comfortable enacting in their lives at the time but rather because it can be seen to also have facilitated encounters between men seeking to enact those fantasies of uninhibited fluid exchanges as the epidemic unfolded. It is the magazine's apparent refusal to stop facilitating raw encounters by censoring those ads that interests me here.

Raw, unprocessed food has historically been seen as a potential source of danger in Western culture. Its mediation through cooking has come to be seen not only as a form of hygiene and therefore prophylaxis, but also for that reason as a sign of civilizational development that reproduced colonial ideologies of European supremacy vis-à-vis non-Western and pre-modern cultures (Lévi-Strauss 1969; Douglas 2002; Harbottle 2004, 17–28).[1] It is *Projet X*'s embrace of rawness and refusal to hygienize its pages, that makes it stand out from the likes of *Drummer* against which the editors of the French magazine enjoyed comparing themselves by often negatively reviewing issues of their US counterpart as being sexually bland and unadventurous—too cooked, one could say.[2] If *Drummer*, with its growing inclusion of safer-sex pieces and activist op-eds on the epidemic alongside pornographic content, can be seen to have embodied Douglas Crimp's claim that promiscuity would save gay men from HIV by opening us to incorporate condoms into our experimental and open-minded sexual practices, *Projet X*'s direct engagement with AIDS was minimal, leaving it solely up to readers to decide what kinds of sex they would get into, drawing the line purely at the necessity of mutual consent.

Considering the level of detailed didactic information the magazine gave on topics like sex toys, fisting, or bondage techniques, its lack of more substantial engagement with safer sex and the politics of AIDS raises important questions. Assuming that both *Drummer* and *Projet X* catered to a similar readership of gay men into fetish and kink sex scenes, to what extent did the cultural and political specificities of the French gay scene during the 1990s allow for such different approach to the epidemic? What was different about French gay cultures that seem to have complicated Douglas Crimp's earlier claim that with the onset of the AIDS epidemic gay men came together to advocate for safer sex and to join arms against the inertia of politicians, medical researchers, and pharmaceutical companies? Why does AIDS appear to not have straightforwardly been the glue holding French gay men together as a politicized community during the 1990s in the way that it is often assumed thanks to the privileging of US histories of activism in the writing of global histories of homosexuality and the epidemic? Focusing on these questions through the lens of the 1990s in France will allow us to better understand the role played by national political and social contexts in shaping different histories of the gay movement and of its responses to AIDS in the Global North.

FRENCH HOMOSEXUAL ACTIVISM BETWEEN UNIVERSALISM AND COMMUNITARIANISM

By the time what we have come to know as AIDS hit public consciousness in 1981 in the United States, the US and French gay movements could not have been more different. In the United States, the movement had since the 1970s been marked by a politics of identity, publicness, and community liberation. In France, it had tended to frame its politics within a logic of universalism. For Arcadie, the homophile organization founded by André Baudry in 1954, it was universalism of social inclusion and bourgeois respectability. For the FHAR, the radical group founded in 1971, it was a kind of Marxist universalism that saw (homo)sexual liberation as part of the anti-capitalist class struggle against the Oedipal family, the pillar of capital accumulation (Jackson 2009, 4–8; FHAR [1971] 2013). Their radically different political projects notwithstanding, both French homosexual organizations were deeply critical of gay "ghettos" such as commercial enterprises like gay saunas, bars, and clubs, as well as non-commercial ones such as public toilets and outdoors cruising spaces—because they were seen to reduce homosexuality to fleeting sexual encounters, splitting the subject and leaving homosexuals depoliticized, susceptible not only to continued repression but also to ideological and capitalist exploitation (Jackson 2009, 222–225). As the FHAR wrote in response to the visual culture of gay "clone" masculinities that had been emerging in the United States during the 1970s mediated by illustrations by the likes of Tom of Finland:

> Le flic au sexe disproportionné, merveilleusement sanglé dans son uniforme noir et les voyous « à la lourde braguette » sont réconciliés dans le culte du phallus et du trou du cul. Les bandes dessinées pour homosexuels aux États-Unis ou au Danemark sont pleines de ces scènes plus débiles que pornographiques où matons et prisonniers, flics et truands s'entreculent joyeusement dans le meilleur des paradis homosexuels. L'idéologie fasciste tente ainsi de récupérer les

pédés, et il s'en trouve évidemment pour bander devant ces dessins ou photos pleins d'uniformes de cuir et de croix gammées. On voudrait nous faire croire que le nazisme était un paradis pour la pédale, à moins qu'on ne compte sure notre prétendu masochisme. (FHAR 2013 [1971], 48)

[The cop with a disproportionate sex, wonderfully cinched in his black uniform, and the thugs with a large bulge are reconciled in the cult of the phallus and the asshole. Gay comics in the United States and Denmark are full of these scenes, more stupid than pornographic, where guards and prisoners, cops and hoodlums, joyfully fuck each other in the best of gay paradises. Fascist ideology is thus trying to get faggots back, and there are obviously some who get hard in front of these drawings or photos full of leather uniforms and swastikas. They would have us believe that Nazism was a paradise for the faggotry, unless they are taking into account our alleged masochism.]

Despite its critiques of a ghettoized homosexual culture distilled into nothing but sex, despite its framing of homosexual desires and pleasures within the wider context of anti-capitalist and anti-Oedipal political struggles, even the FHAR was looked at with suspicion by the institutionalized French Left such as "Trade unionists, Socialists, Communists, Maoists, or Trotskyists," who considered homosexuality a vice connected to the corruption and decadence of the bourgeoisie (Sibalis 2009, 245). According to the prevailing leftist logics in France at the time, any attempts to split the working classes into special interest groups like identity "communities" could only corrupt class consciousness and thus pose a threat to both class struggle and the cohesion of the proletariat understood as the universal agent of history's unfolding. Such a view of politics was not restricted to Left orthodoxy, however. Instead, suspicion of special interest group politics was widespread in the French political landscape where "the prevailing republican tradition of egalitarianism and universalism [conflicted] with the pursuit of a specific group identity and the representation of particular desires and interests" (Fillieule and Duyvendak 1999, 185). With narratives of political universalism sustaining the mythology of the Fifth Republic and of its institutions, even the events of May 1968 at the Sorbonne, with their questioning of tradition, authority and sexual morality having opened the way for the appearance of the FHAR in 1971, can at best only be seen, retrospectively, as a "'moral revolution,' . . . not a political or social one" (Sibalis 2009, 236). As David Caron (1998) noted, "the republican model needs to construct a homogenous other against which to define itself and hide its internal contradictions. . . . Hence the tendency in France today to have the words *républicanisme* and *communautarisme* followed by *à la française* or *à l'américaine* respectively" (285). This ideological divide between republicanism and communitarianism, which developed in France to protect the origin myth of a singular and universal French republic would eventually be institutionalized even further with the election of François Mitterrand in 1981, the same year the US Centers for Disease Control (CDC) first announced the deaths of otherwise "healthy" homosexual men due to *pneumocystis pneumonia*, later found to have been triggered by immunodeficiency due to HIV infection (CDC 1981).

THE PRIVATE AND THE PUBLIC IN FRENCH AIDS ACTIVISM

With many noted French intellectuals like Guy Hocquenghem, Michel Foucault, Simone de Beauvoir, Gilles Deleuze, or Félix Guattari having urged gay men to vote for Mitterrand's Socialist Party (Martel 1999, 127), the legal status of homosexuals in France changed rapidly in the aftermath of the 1981 election. While consensual same-sex activity had been legal in France since 1791 when the Constituent Assembly repealed anti-sodomy laws (Sibalis 1996, 80), the collaborationist Vichy government of Marshal Pétain had later reintroduced a legal distinction between "natural" and "unnatural" sexual acts which criminalized same-sex acts between an adult and a minor under twenty-one while the age of consent for heterosexual acts was set at thirteen. After World War II and the French Liberation, the provisional government of Charles de Gaulle kept Pétain's distinction in law, reaffirming the age of consent for homosexual acts at twenty-one while raising it to fifteen for heterosexual ones (Sibalis 1996, 84–85; 231). It was not until 1982 with the homosexual coalition Comité d'Urgence Anti-Répression Homosexuelle (Urgency Committee Against the Repression of Homosexuals), also known as CUARH, having taken on the role of mediator between French homosexuals and the newly-appointed cabinet led by Mitterrand that the new Socialist-majority National Assembly voted in favor of the abrogation of paragraph 2 of article 331 of the Penal Code—the one that had lingered since Pétain—therefore equalizing the age of consent and signaling a political convergence of the French state and the French homosexual movement.

As such, after the first cases of AIDS were identified in the United States in 1981, French intellectuals within and without the gay movement responded with suspicion to the news (Dodier 2003). First, this response was due to the movement's resistance against what was perceived to be a renewed attack on the sexual freedoms that had been fought for and gained since the 1970s, of which the election of François Mitterrand that same year and the subsequent equalization of the age of consent would become the latest examples (Martel 1999, 187–215; Broqua 2005, 20–21). Second, in a country like France where Republican ideology required a dialectical tension between the universalism posited for and by the state and the particularism attributed to communities

(Caron 1998), recognizing a new "disease" which seemed to discriminate specific segments of the population would call into question "the pre-existing conceptions and certainties of the nation's self-narration" (Pratt 2012, 184). As a result, and unlike countries like the United States where the AIDS organization Gay Men's Health Crisis (GMHC) was founded in 1982 and partly responsible for what Crimp (1987) saw as the gay grassroots "invention" of safer-sex practices (253), the climate in France during the first years of the epidemic was marked by community inaction and political deadlocks which, in Caron's words (1998), reflected "a tension inherent in the construction of homosexuality in modern French culture, where the homosexual is at the same time an individual citizen with a right to his private sex life, and a distinct and despised species." As a result, "gay identity, it seems, [did] and [did] not exist as a working category in French society" (286).

France would therefore have to wait until 1984, when Daniel Defert founded AIDES in the aftermath of the death of his partner Michel Foucault, to have an AIDS organization capable of raising awareness, supporting patients, effectively lobbying politicians, and carrying out work within communities. However, unlike the GMHC in the United States, AIDES never positioned itself straightforwardly as a homosexual interest organization (Dodier 2003; Girard 2016). The first decade of the epidemic in France was thus marked by what Christophe Broqua (2005) describes as "une épidémie à deux visages: dans les discours officiels, une maladie concernant indistinctement l'ensemble de la population: dans l'expérience direct du sida, une épidémie cantonnée aux homosexuels et aux usagers de drogues" ["an epidemic with two speeds and two faces: in official discourse, a disease that concerned the whole population indistinctly; in direct experiences of AIDS, an epidemic confined to homosexuals and drug users"] (19). The result was therefore that throughout the early 1980s, the French fight against the epidemic was marked by an elevation of AIDS to the status of a general public health issue, thanks to a convergence of medical-scientific institutions with the universalist ideologies of the Republic, in that "la circulation dans l'espace public d'une information cohérente, unifiée, et contrôlée par les institutions scientifiques, est considérée comme un outil indispensable pour s'opposer, grâce à la raison, aux attitudes et aux pratiques de stigmatization, celles-ci étant considérées, du point de vue de l'option moderne-libérale, comme un comportement irrationnel" ["the circulation in the public sphere of coherent, unified information controlled by scientific institutions is taken to be an indispensable tool to oppose, through reason, stigmatizing attitudes and practices, which are considered, from the viewpoint of modern liberalism, as irrational behaviors"] (Dodier 2003, 2). Yet, at the same time, on the ground, new organizations started emerging that worked primarily with specific populations due to a sense that their needs were not being addressed. In the case of some French gay activists who had been watching their peers become the face of AIDS activism and lobbying in the United States, the shortcomings of the French strategy to fight AIDS—with France having come second to the United States in numbers of cases in the Global North—were due, first, to what was largely seen as a dissolution of the gay movement in the aftermath of Mitterrand's 1981 election (Caron 1998; Poulin-Deltour 2004) and, second, to the perceived "dehomosexualisation of AIDS" at the hands of French institutions and organizations like AIDES (Ernst 1997; Broqua 2005). It was that realization of the shortcomings of the official French response to AIDS that eventually led to the formation of ACT UP Paris in 1989, modelled on its New York counterpart that had been founded two years prior.

Appearing as the result of an eventual—that is, late—awareness among French gay men that AIDS was real and primarily affecting male homosexual communities, the formation of ACT UP Paris in 1989 also signaled a change in the public perception of the epidemic away from being a matter of public interest toward it being first and foremost a matter of community concern. As Cristophe Broqua (2005) notes, "Act Up va rendre possible un nécessaire travail de mise en cohérence de l'expérience de l'homosexualité avec celle du sida, tant au niveau individual qu'au niveau collectif" ["Act Up would make possible the necessary work of making homosexual experience and the experience of AIDS coherent with one another, both at the individual and collective level"] (22). To do this, ACT UP Paris would be responsible for constructing and promoting a wholly new political actor in the French social and cultural landscape, that of the HIV-positive homosexual. Through that strategy, the organization not only politicized AIDS but also, and most importantly, placed AIDS at the center of French homosexual identity which, as a consequence, would itself become politicized for the first time since the 1970s. ACT UP's strategy therefore involved, first, the reactivation of a homosexual politics around AIDS. Secondly, it involved the construction and advocacy of a new form of homosexual militant identity that would make public—that is, political—matters theretofore restricted to the private sphere. Finally, and most importantly, the organization would become the self-appointed spokesperson for French homosexuals, a role that would lead to its own policing of homosexual behaviors. This approach would eventually make them clash with more pragmatic AIDS organizations built on a service model of which AIDES was the biggest representative (Broqua 2005). As a result, in a country whose modern mythic origin story imbued its national identity with idealized visions of equality, universalism, and the public good, the appearance of a new militant AIDS organization foregrounding homosexual lives and experiences of the epidemic ended up seen by many as a threat to the French "republican model of nationhood [which] defines French citizenship as a contract resulting from a political will, from the convergence of free, individual decisions to live together according to a core of basic universal principles" (Caron 1998, 283). In foregrounding not only the political nature of the AIDS crisis but also the limitations of the French official response to the crisis, however, the creation of ACT UP Paris reveals, in a very material way, that the dialectical tension between universalism and communitarianism that had been deployed in national Republican discourse as a way of forging the myth of French singularity vis-à-vis nations such as the United States was also, in fact, fundamentally inherent to the Republic itself. Nowhere would this tension become more visible than at the heart of homosexual and AIDS activism in France, both caught in the vortex created by republican ideologies of *equality* and universal equal rights, and community demands for political autonomy and recognition of their *difference* (Prearo 2014, 300).

PROJET X: HOMOSEXUALITY, PRIVACY, AND CONSENT

It was in this context of tension between two seemingly contradictory and yet co-dependent models of citizenship and political life—one that positioned sexuality and identity at the heart of its political rhetoric, another that restricted them to the private sphere of individuals—that *Projet X* first appeared in 1995 with an editorial line at odds with the public militant model of homosexual identity espoused by ACT UP Paris. Because of that editorial approach, the magazine helps us paint a more complex picture not only of homosexuality vis-à-vis AIDS activism throughout the 1990s in France but also of a certain mythologization of the role played by the AIDS crisis in shaping contemporary homosexual identities, one that continues to be reproduced to this day in popular histories and contemporary forms of AIDS "retroactivism" (Ledin 2021) and political nostalgia.

One telling example of the ways in which the magazine upheld the value of the private/public divide can be found in its coverage of the legal and political aftermath of the infamous Operation Spanner, which had seen several gay and bisexual men arrested and interrogated by the UK's Greater Manchester Police for involvement in consensual sadomasochistic sex, and sixteen of them eventually being charged with several offenses including assault resulting in bodily harm, unlawful wounding, and aiding and abetting assaults against themselves. The men were trialed at the Old Bailey in 1990 (*Regina v. Brown*) and eight of them were given prison sentences. In the following years, some of the convicted appealed to the Court of Appeal, the House of Lords, and finally in 1997 the European Court of Human Rights (*Laskey, Jaggard and Brown v. The United Kingdom*), all of which rejected their appeals.

Unlike AIDS, which had been ravaging the gay community and triggered the re-emergence of public homosexual militancy in France at the hands of ACT UP Paris, the aftermath of the UK's Spanner Case was the single political issue to have ever been covered by *Projet X*. For instance, in issue 2 (December 1995) a piece entitled "Grande-Bretagne: Countdown on Spanner—L'État sadique" (Dodier 2003, 2) ["Great Britain: Countdown on Spanner—The Sadistic State")] claims that despite its long history of accepting corporal punishment as pedagogical tool for children, the Spanner case highlighted the UK's refusal to grant individuals the right to do whatever they wished with their own bodies even in private settings (36). Spanner appeared again in issue 12 (October 1996) as the appeal to the European Court of Human Rights was unfolding. In a text entitled "Le cas Spanner: une issue décisive" ["The Spanner Case: a decisive issue"] which followed coverage of the 1996 SM Pride in London, the author going by the penname Bâtard 28 writes that "l'enjeu n'est ni plus ni moins que la reconnaissance de pouvoir disposer librement de son corps pour le plaisir, quel qu'il soit, *en marquant clairement la frontière entre vie privée et agissements publics*" ["what is at stake is nothing more, nothing less than the recognition of one's ability to freely dispose of one's body for pleasure, whatever it may be, *by clearly marking the boundary between private life and public affairs*"] (43, my emphasis).

The magazine's insistence on the value of the public/private divide as *the* guarantor of (homo)sexual freedoms exemplifies a model of homosexual life in dialectical opposition both with public homosexual activism and with critiques of the public/private divide carried out by queer and feminist US scholars such as Nancy Fraser (1992) or Lauren Berlant and Michael Warner (1998). In their essay "Sex in Public" for instance, Berlant and Warner enacted a critique of the ways in which a Habermasian universalist model of the polity (Habermas 1991) segregates the sexual lives of subjects and therefore their different sexual cultures from the forms of citizenship it values as pillars of political life. It does so by confining sexuality to the realm of private life and by removing it from the public sphere where the politics it both idealizes and regulates takes place. As such, the authors argue that universalist models of public and thus political life fail to account for the ways in which queer forms of intimacy "bear no necessary relation to domestic space, to kinship, to the couple form, to property, or to the nation" (Berlant and Warner 1998, 558).

Projet X inhabited, from its beginnings in 1995, a space that complicates the above critiques of the public/private divide and, therefore, of the value of publicness in queer lives and politics. That is clear not only from its valorization of the right to privacy as the single guarantor of sexual freedom, but also from the editorial line it adopted vis-à-vis AIDS, one that, as I have already argued, refused to hygienize the pages of the magazine, leaving it solely up to its readers to decide the risks they would be willing to take. The magazine's relationship with the community activists and its spokespersons was, therefore, not without tension—much to the contrary. The overtly political editorial signed by "Dick" (François Agrapart) that opened the bilingual issue 22 (September 1997)—a telling exception in the history of a magazine that has otherwise seldom made political pronouncements—is a case in point, hinting at the tensions within a gay community marked by internal ideological fractures:

> Here and there in the "community" press that pretends to represent "ideal" gay life, politically correct, cultivated, elegant, humorous (often bitchy) and where the only eccentricity allowed is a certain non-vulgar campness (except on Saturday nights), there have recently been some statements that are astonishing considering the clichés of tolerance that abound as far as so-called "gay solidarity" is concerned.
>
> Hard queers have been represented as freaks by the comparison of fist fucking with emptying out a chicken (Têtu), by the opinion that most of us have dangerous sexual activities (Têtu again), and by the idea that we all read controversial literature like Projet X . . . (Ex-Aequo),
>
> May we remind all these people who have embraced the idea that homosexuality is acquiring a certain social acceptance that the ideals that they once defended (with us) are still valid for all of us.
>
> There is no division to be made between "uncontrollable SM queers" (even though I find such a tag appealing) and "clean, nice homosexuals." The number of people that drift somewhere in the middle between these two categories with more or less hard, extreme and fetishist practices is so vast that any idea of two opposing groups is ridiculous.
>
> As if inserting one, two or three fingers in a guy's arse is correct, the fourth signals the danger line of debauchery and with the fifth you become politically incorrect?
>
> A piercing is cool if it's to wear out to a club, but not if it's used within sexual activity?
>
> Is this social dynamics expressing itself? Is this a group of once outcasts integrating society and in doing so relegating some of their brothers to the role of scapegoat to strengthen their feeling of belonging to society?
>
> Perhaps it is logical and useful to some gay media to try to portray us as the black sheep of the affair . . . (1)

The pages of *Projet X*, from its first to its last issue, offer a valuable subcultural snapshot of the dialectical tensions between private identities and public militancy at the heart of the French gay movement and AIDS activism as the

21st century was dawning. They reveal in a very tangible and raw manner the ways in which gay male responses to AIDS—or lack thereof—during the first decades of the epidemic cannot be exhausted by extant historical and critical discourses that have tended to portray a homogenous gay "community" united behind the banner of AIDS activism and "safe sex." In highlighting the limitations of straightforwardly extending geographically specific narratives of AIDS politics and homosexual activism from national to so-called "global" contexts, *Projet X* and its content I have discussed here also raise important and timely questions about existing AIDS historiography, and about taken-for-granted views of the crisis and of gay men's engagement in activism. These questions become all the more pressing in the context of contemporary AIDS revisitation media narratives which continue in large part to anchor their stories in the figures of either activists or a generalized politicized "community." Granted, narratives such as those had their political valences in the early years of the epidemic, such as when Douglas Crimp tied the now canonical knot between gay promiscuity and safe sex with "How to Have Promiscuity in an Epidemic" (1987). They helped gay men push back against a growing stigmatization of their lives and sex cultures triggered by AIDS panic. The flipside of that, however, is that the ethical complexities of gay men's sex lives during those last decades of the 20th century became subsumed by narratives that, willfully or not, ended up being part of a wider project of homosexual atonement and redemption in the years that followed the public onset of AIDS. Veering away from the privileging of activist actors in the writing of gay histories and toward broader gay male cultures of consumption and subcultural media allows us to get a better grasp of the complexities and internal tensions of a gay "community" well beyond activist paradigms and political allegiances. In the case of France and *Projet X* in particular, such an approach helps us get a clearer sense of the ways in which a dialectics of both universalism and communitarianism, and public and private, was not only the engine of France's own nationalist mythology and homosexual politics, but that it also played itself out in arguably the most unlikely of places—the pages of a magazine created and sold with the sole purpose of getting gay men off.

BIBLIOGRAPHY

Andersson, Johan. 2018. "Homonormative Aesthetics: AIDS and 'De-Generational Unremembering' in 1990s London." *Urban Studies* 56 (14): 2993–3010.

Berlant, Lauren, and Michael Warner. 1998. "Sex in Public." *Critical Inquiry* 24 (2): 547–566.

Broqua, Christophe. 2005. *Agir Pour Ne Pas Mourir! Act Up, Les Homosexuels et le SIDA*. Paris: Presses de Sciences Po.

Caron, David. 1998. "*Liberté, Égalité, Séroposivité*: AIDS, the French Republic, and the Question of Community." *French Cultural Studies* 9 (27): 281–293.

Cascais, António Fernando. 2006. "Diferentes Como Só Nós: O Associativismo GLBT Português em Três Andamentos." *Revista Crítica de Ciências Sociais* 76: 109–126.

Castiglia, Christopher, and Christopher Reed. 2012. *If Memory Serves: Gay Men, AIDS, and the Promise of the Queer Past*. Minneapolis: University of Minnesota Press.

CDC. 1981. "Epidemiologic Notes and Reports: *Pneumocystis* Pneumonia—Los Angeles." *Morbidity and Mortality Weekly Report* 30 (21): 1–3.

Cheng, Jih-Fei, Alexandra Juhasz, and Nishant Shahani. 2020. "Introduction." In *AIDS and the Distribution of Crises*, edited by Jih-Fei Cheng, Alexandra Juhasz, and Nishant Shahani, 1–28. Durham: Duke University Press.

Crimp, Douglas. 1987. "How to Have Promiscuity in an Epidemic." *October* 43: 237–271.

Davis, Oliver. 2015. "Leading by Example: A Queer Critique of Personalization and Coercive Community Governance in Act Up-Paris's Operation Against Bareback Writers." *Sexualities* 18 (1/2): 141–157.

Dodier, Nicolas. 2003. "Les Premières Années de l'Épidemie de SIDA et la Conversion Politique du Mouvement Homosexuel." In *Homosexualités au Temps du SIDA: Tensions Sociales et Identitaires*, edited by Christophe Broqua, France Lert, and Yves Souteyrand, 1–18. Paris: Agence Nationale de Recherches sur le SIDA.

Douglas, Mary. 2002. *Purity and Danger: An Analysis of Concept of Pollution and Taboo*. New York: Routledge.

Ernst, Claire E. 1997. "Activisme à l'Américaine? The Case of Act Up Paris." *French Politics and Society* 15 (4): 22–31.

FHAR. 2013. *Rapport Contre la Normalité*. Montpellier: GayKitschCamp.

Fillieule, Olivier, and Jan Willem Duyvendak. 1999. "Gay and Lesbian Activism in France: Between Integration and Community-Oriented Movements." In *The Global Emergence of Gay and Lesbian Politics: National Imprints of a Worldwide Movement*, edited by Barry D. Adam, Jan Willem Duyvedak, and André Krouwel, 184–213. Phliladelphia: Temple University Press.

Florêncio, João. 2020. *Bareback Porn, Porous Masculinities, Queer Futures: The Ethics of Becoming-Pig*. Abingdon: Routledge.

Fraser, Nancy. 1992. "Rethinking the Public Sphere: A Contribution to the Critique of Actually Existing Democracy." In *Habermas and the Public Sphere*, edited by Craig Calhoun, 109–142. Cambridge, MA: The MIT Press.

Freeman, Richard. 1992. "Governing the Voluntary Sector Response to AIDS: A Comparative Study of the UK and Germany." *Voluntas* 3 (1): 29–47.

Girard, Gabriel. 2014. "Les Controverses sur le Risque du SIDA chez les Gays et la Question de la Normalisation de l'Homosexualité." *Hermès* 69: 160–162.

Girard, Gabriel. 2016. "VIH/SIDA, l'Épidémie qui a Révolutionné la Sexualité?" *Rhizome: Bulletin National Santé Mentale et Précarité* 60: 5–6.

Habermas, Jürgen. 1991. *The Structural Transformation of the Public Sphere: An Inquiry into a Category of Bourgeois Society*. Cambridge, MA: The MIT Press.

Halkitis, Perry. 2000. "Masculinity in the Age of AIDS: HIV-Seropositive Gay Men and the 'Buff Agenda.'" In *Gay Masculinities*, edited by Peter Nardi, 130–151. Thousand Oaks, CA: Sage Publications.

Harbottle, Lynn. 2004. *Food for Health, Food for Wealth: Ethnic and Gender Identities in British Iranian Communities*. New York: Berghahn Books.

Haus, Sebastian. 2016. "Risky Sex—Risky Language. HIV/AIDS and the West German Gay Scene in the 1980s." *Historical Social Research/Historische Sozial-forschung* 41 (1): 111–134.

Hilderbrand, Lucas. 2006. "Retroactivism." *GLQ* 12 (2): 303–317.

Jackson, Julian. 2009. *Living in Arcadia: Homosexuality, Politics, and Morality in France from the Liberation to AIDS*. Chicago: The University of Chicago Press.

Johnson, David K. 2019. *Buying Gay: How Physique Entrepreneurs Sparked a Movement*. New York: Columbia University Press.

Lecklider, Aaron S. 2021. *Love's Next Meeting: The Forgotten History of Homosexuality and the Left in American Culture*. Oakland: University of California Press.

Ledin, Chase. 2021. "Retroactivism and Futurity in *120BPM*." *Modern and Contemporary France*. Special Issue: "Robin Campillo's *120BPM* (2017): Screening AIDS, Activism, and Queer Identity in Contemporary France. Typeset manuscript. Forthcoming.

Lévi-Strauss, Claude. 1969. *The Raw and the Cooked: Introduction to a Science of Mythology, I*. New York: Harper & Row.

Maron, Dina. 2020. "'Wet Markets Likely Launched the Coronavirus. Here's What You Need to Know." *National Geographic*, 16 April 2020. https://www.nationalgeographic.co.uk/science-and-technology/2020/04/wet-markets-likely-launched-coronavirus-heres-what-you-need-know [accessed 10 October 2021].

Martel, Frédéric. 1999. *The Pink and the Black: Homosexuals in France since 1968*. Stanford: Stanford University Press.

Meyer, Richard. 2003. "The Jesse Helms Theory of Art." *October* 104: 131–148.

Poulin-Deltour, William J. 2004. "French Gay Activism and the American Referent in Contemporary France." *The French Review* 78 (1): 118–125.

Pratt, Murray. 2012. "Getting It from Noise and Other Myths: AIDS and Intellectuals in France." *Paragraph* 35 (2): 181–196.

Prearo, Massimo. 2014. *Le Moment Politique de l'Homosexualité: Mouvements, Identités et Communautés en France*. Lyon: Presses Universitaires de Lyon.

Richardson, Diane. 2005. "Desiring Sameness? The Rise of a Neoliberal Politics of Normalisation." *Antipode* 37 (3): 515–535.

Schulman, Sarah. 2012. *The Gentrification of the Mind: Witness to a Lost Imagination*. Berkeley: University of California Press.

Schulman, Sarah. 2021. *Let The Record Show: A Political History of Act Up New York, 1987–1993*. New York: Farrar, Straus and Giroux.

Shepard, Benjamin. 2001. "The Queer/Gay Assimilationist Split: The Suits vs. the Sluts." *Monthly Review* 53 (1): 49–62.

Sibalis, Michael, 1996. "The Regulation of Male Homosexuality in Revolutionary and Napoleonic France, 1789–1815." In *Homosexuality in Modern France*, edited by Jeffrey Merrick, and Bryant T. Ragan, Jr., 80–101. New York: Oxford University Press.

Sibalis, Michael. 2009. "The Spirit of May '68 and the Origins of the Gay Liberation Movement in France." In *Gender and Sexuality in 1968: Transformative Politics in the Cultural Imagination*, edited by Lessie Jo Frazier, and Deborah Cohen, 235–253. New York: Palgrave Macmillan.

Warner, Michael. 2009. "Unsafe: Why Gay Men Are Having Risky Sex." In David M. Halperin, *What Do Gay Men Want? An Essay on Sex, Risk, and Subjectivity*, 157–169. Ann Arbor: The University of Michigan Press.

Xiao Xiao et al. 2021. "Animal Sales from Wuhan Wet Markets Immediately Prior to the COVID-19 Pandemic." *Nature Scientific Reports* 11: 11898.

NOTES

1. The most recent example of this framing of rawness as taboo and vector of infection can be seen in the very public popular and scientific debates that have been ongoing in the context of the COVID-19 pandemic on whether SARS-CoV-2 may have been passed from animals to humans at the "exotic" wet markets of Wuhan, China (Maron 2020; Xiao Xiao et al. 2021).

2. Examples of *Projet X*'s scathing reviews of *Drummer* can be found in issue 7 (May, 1996), where it is claimed that *Drummer* is becoming "more and more sanitised" (46). In the following issue—issue 8 (June, 1996)—the US magazine is written about as being "in a slump" ["*dans un passage à vide*"] and "completely uninteresting" ["*carrément sans intérêt*"], while in issue 20 (June, 1997), a bilingual review repeats the claim, also seen in most other *Projet X* reviews of *Drummer* 202, that it is basically made up of "the usual fodder of studio photos (yawn), and images that we've already seen over the last few months" (56).

Chapter Six

Viral Dances

Moving in Times of a Pandemic

Lucille Toth

Epidemics and pandemics have fascinated all forms of literature and arts; they have also led to the production of a rich scholarship. Nevertheless, dance remains academically less explored in its relationship to contamination, especially in the French context.[1] In April 2021, I was invited to join the jury of the WE-Program[2], an international dance project led by Mathilde Gilhet that aims to provide virtual, low-cost dance education and offers an award to one emerging mover each month. Among all the applications—180 in total—80 percent were about the impact of COVID-19 on the life and creative process of the applicants. Many of them raised similar issues: How can one create while physically and mentally isolated? How can one rethink the geographies of dance in order to develop solo pieces instead of larger ensembles? These questions speak volumes to the ways in which epidemics have historically impacted movements and reshaped dance.

This chapter aims to focus on three key moments in the history of viral dances: the Saint Vitus' dancing plagues in 16th-century France, 1990s HIV+ performers dancing, and TikTok viral dances during the ongoing COVID-19 pandemic. Each of these moments has produced new discourses on contagion and movement and shows the importance of reading dance through the medical humanities. The Saint Vitus' dancing plagues implemented a new vision of dance as a possible contaminating agent through an invisible infectiousness. HIV+ dancers used dance as a healing therapy for what I will call a generational kinesthetic trauma. Today, with COVID-19, viral dance is redefining the geographies of dance thanks to digital tools. By investigating these three key moments together, my goal is to propose a better understanding of the political roles of dance when using a raw aesthetic. In the context of pandemics, raw aesthetics in dance challenge a canonical glorious and athletic body, created to insure bienséance and harmony.[3] I argue that viral dance generates cultural productions that foreground the transhistorical perspectives of dance and contamination insofar as choreographic art allows an unaesthetic, raw, sick body to enter the public space.

Confronting dance with the idea of virality necessitates reevaluating the place of viral discourses in today's field of French studies and investigating how pandemics push scholars and practitioners toward intellectual creativity and activism. Looking to other epidemics provides key lessons to better understand HIV/AIDS and the historical porosity between pandemics. It seems impossible to experience COVID-19 without looking back to the knowledge gained by the research on HIV/AIDS, the cultural and social structures put in place, and the ways pandemics affect marginalized bodies through their policing.

SAINT VITUS' DANCE: FIRST VIRAL MOVEMENT

In the beginning of the 13th century, outbreaks of dancing mania, as 16th-century Swiss physicist Paracelse named it, and other delirious behaviors emerged in most of Europe, the most famous of which occurred in Strasbourg, France, on July 14, 1518. This event was known as Saint Vitus' dance—Vitus being the patron saint of neurological disorders—as well as Sydenham chorea, as 17th-century British physician Thomas Sydenham later named it. DC Schecter writes:

> Saint Vitus' dance is a sort of convulsion which attacks boys and girls from the tenth year till they have done growing. At first it shows itself by a halting, or rather an unsteady movement of one of the legs, which the patient drags. Then it is seen in the hand of the same side. The patient cannot keep it a moment in its place, whether he lay it upon his breast or any other part of his body. Do what he may, it will be jerked elsewhere convulsively. (1975, 1091–1102)

Frau Troffea was the first known case of this malady and, "to the consternation of her husband, went on dancing throughout the day . . . Only after many hours of crazed motion did she collapse from exhaustion. Bathed in sweat and with muscles twitching, she finally sank into a brief restorative sleep. Then, a few hours later, she resumed her solitary jig" (Waller 2009, 1). Frau Troffea was not the first "manic" dancer in the history of viral dance. However, she was the first to launch an epidemic with more than five hundred people joining the dance. "Within days, more than thirty people had taken to the streets, seized by the same urgent need to dance, hop, and leap into the air . . . By the early August 1518, the epidemic had begun to spread at an alarming rate . . . Exactly how many fell dead we cannot know, though one chronicle suggests that (at least for a time) fifteen were dying each day as they danced in the punishing summer heat, seldom pausing to eat, drink, or rest" (3). Between the fourteenth and fifteenth centuries, these epidemics were inscribed in the collective memory through various medieval chronicles[4] and have endured in the collective imagination for their crude aesthetic so much so that one could argue that dance can be perceived as a threatening art which can trigger epidemics not through a viral contamination but rather an invisible contaminating effect.

The fascination for viral dance lasted for centuries and inspired many artists. Pieter Brueghel the Elder famously depicts them in 1564 in a well-known print entitled "Procession of the Possessed"; the English rock band Bauhaus's 1980s song clearly refers to "St Vitus Dance"; and in 2018, French writer Jean Teulé's *Entrez dans la danse* imagines the city of Strasbourg's efforts to heal ill-stricken people to restore order to the city.

To date, we can only speculate on the origin and reasons behind the Saint Vitus' chorea. For Paracelse, these dancing manias are clear revolts perpetrated by women who are fighting against the constraints of married life. For 19th-century German medical writer Justus Hecker, the accounts of medieval dance epidemics are colored with a moralizing lexicon that is similar to that of the Christian Middle Ages. For him, the dance mania can spread and infect through the sight of the sick, as if it is a "demoniacal epidemic over the whole of Germany and the neighboring countries to the north-west, which [are] already prepared for its reception by the prevailing opinions of the times" (Hecker 2020, 106). The juxtaposition of Christian and medical signifiers in the phrase "demonical epidemic" reveals a tension between two traditions of knowledge "illuminating the original ties between medicine and religious mysticism and highlighting major breakthroughs in the advancement of medicine, including the germ theory and biological psychiatry" (Bonthius and Karacay 2003, 11). The Christian ideology would consider the rawness of this dance as evil. Its natural, unprocessed, and violent state challenged the power structure imposed by religious institutions in order to civilize and control citizens with Christian values.

Even though the clinical definition of a virus in its modern understanding will only appear in the 19th century, it is important to capture the impact of the spectacle that was Saint Vitus' dance on the imaginary of contamination as it pertains specifically to its legacy in the following centuries. Hecker dedicated three chapters to this dancing plague in his study *The Epidemics of the Middle Ages*. He describes Saint Vitus' dancers as such: "Those affected fell to the ground senseless, panting and laboring for breath. They foamed at the mouth, and suddenly springing up began their dance amidst strange contortions"

(2020, 100). The primitive aspect of this dance, the lack of bodily control, the physical dejections (foam, sweat) seem reminiscent of Jean-Martin Charcot's depictions of hysteria. As the director of the Salpêtrière Asylum in Paris in the mid-19th century, Charcot made hysteria "an object of public spectacle" (Stephenson 2001, 27) as "the seizures of hysterical patients are presented in Charcot's auditorium during his famous lessons, and the performativity of the body in pain is photographically immortalized" (Perreault 2020, 49). Charcot developed a theatricalization of hysteria: "He would hypnotize his female 'hysterics' so as to trigger fits during which they would spasm, hallucinate, and convulse, become mute or lose sensation, while their limbs became twisted and contorted, and some collapsed to the floor with their spines, arms, and heads curved backward toward their feet in what was called the *arc de cercle*." (Waller 2009, 219) Nevertheless, beyond the neurological explanation of Charcot, an agency was fantasized. Similarly to Paracelse's idea that Saint Vitus' female dancers resisted domestic life through their contortions, Charcot's patients stand as a figure of resistance to what Foucault named "psychiatric power," that is to say a "supplement of power by which the real is imposed on madness in the name of a truth held once and for all by this power under the name of medical science, psychiatry" (2003, 61–62). Suffering from seizures, convulsions, and other movements that resemble Saint Vitus' dance, the patients were psychiatrized and placed within a system of domination of medical power. Resistance was made possible by the reappropriation of a stolen voice in the production of a discourse of truth.

The question of the spectacle brings to the fore the question of the audience and its hierarchy. Who is watching (and judging) Frau Troffea's foam escaping her mouth while in trance? Who is watching (and enjoying) the spectacle of the Salpêtrière women's contortions during their epileptic-like crisis? The hierarchy in this spectacle is clear. The sick are watched by the non-sick: Frau Troffea is watched by the city's authorities who want to restore order, and the Salpêtrière's women are watched by the masculine, medical gaze. A century later, gay HIV+ patients will be watched by the straight majority. When the AIDS epidemic was called "the gay disease," it put the blame only on one specific marginal group. Similarly, even though neither hysteria nor Saint Vitus' dance only concerned women, they are the most portrayed in visual and literary archives on manic dances. Waller argues that "since low-status women in many cultures have had poorer diets than their husbands, this may help explain why they are usually overrepresented among those suffering from spontaneous trances" (2009, 206). The very concept of 'patient zero' speaks volumes to the ways discourses of pandemics create a hierarchy, allowing for blaming minorities and reinforcing a moral need of "othering." One infamous instance of the patient zero narrative, for instance, was Irish immigrant Mary Mallon, otherwise known as "Typhoid Mary," who was accused of spreading typhoid through her cooking. In 1907, "about 3,000 New Yorkers had been infected by *Salmonella typhi*, and probably Mary was the main reason for the outbreak" (Filio et al. 2013, 132–134). Another patient zero myth was that of flight attendant Gaétan Dugas,[5] an immigrant and openly gay man who became the face of the AIDS epidemic and of gay sexual behaviors as he was conveniently blamed for the spread of the virus.[6] Was Frau Troffea another convenient first known case in the way that such a status continued to fuel a long-lasting project of medical power over powerless bodies?

Regardless of the era, epidemics affect marginalized communities and vulnerable voiceless people in ways that go beyond the medical concern. Pre-established social stigmas allow public discourse to shame and accuse minorities to hold them responsible. This issue leads us to rethinking the collective form of dance as it continues to pose a threat to social equilibrium and to a historical, authoritarian system of beliefs. With the AIDS epidemic, healing dance, both collective and individual, will develop to oppose discourses of social threat and stigma.

AIDS: HEALING DANCE

> A large pile of boxes neatly stacked in front of him, Alain Buffard crouches down and sticks one of the tubes of Retrovir on a very long white plaster. He then peels it off from its protective tab with the accompanying tearing noise and sticks the whole thing to his heel. He repeats this ritual for the other leg. Tube under heel. Tape. Noise. Glue. Once the Retrovir heels are created, he takes the pile of boxes in his hands, stands up and begins walking on Kevin Coyne's song *Good Boy*. Like a fashion show, he stops his walk from time to time and poses in front of the audience. As he walks around, the boxes fall down, and the stack crumbles. Ultimately, it's the heels that break. Alain Buffard stops, turning his back to the public. He leans forward, barefoot.[7]

This scene comes from the solo piece *Good Boy*, created and performed by HIV+ French movement artist Alain Buffard in 1998 at La Ménagerie de Verre in Paris, France. The elegant-heeled walk of Buffard sets his body in motion, a body which can stand upright, walk, and function thanks to new medication. Deeply transformed by the arrival of new drugs such as Retrovil, Buffard's walk is inscribed in a particular temporality: "After the use of AZT as monotherapy from 1986, it took four years to start treatments combining two drugs such as AZT and 3TC . . . This dual therapy has shown its superiority over previous monotherapies and paved the way for more effective treatments. Treatment for the virus was still partial, but significant nonetheless: while AZT gave a four-to-six-month reprieve, it was reduced to one year"

(Routy 2011, 117). It is not so much the staging of the dying body that matters to Buffard in this scene, rather, it is an intimate reflection on the state of his medicated viral body which must remain constantly in a state of vigilance.

Good Boy is the first part of a triptych, followed by the quartet *Good For . . .* (2001) and the group piece *Mauvais Genre* (2004). François Frimat refers to this triptych as "a centrifugal movement, delegating to more and more other bodies the care of experimenting with the material of the solo, like a propagation by contagion, like the disease that works the body in question here" (2011, 96). In *Mauvais Genre*'s note of intent, Buffard explains: "Je voulais voir ce que donneraient, transposées à d'autres corps, chacun porteur d'une histoire individuelle, les propositions de ce premier travail" ["I wanted to see what the propositions from this first piece, once applied to other bodies and each carrying an individual story, would yield"] (Buffard). The forty dancers walk in an arrogant demeanor. They are proud to be on the heels of Retrovil. They pose in the middle of the audience, yet the dancers are not the only ones who have to walk. The audience is also invited to take a stroll with them. François Frimat explains that "as a spectator, we find ourselves becoming actor of the climate that is setting in, as well as co-author of the collective situation created" (2011, 99). Even if the audience is not carrying Retrovil boxes, they become part of the collective, viral story.

In *My Lunch with Anna* (2005), choreographer Anna Halprin is in dialogue with Buffard. They are filmed having lunch in San Francisco, and it is during these scenes that Buffard explains that he discovered his HIV+ status in 1988. It is in this moment when he decides to stop dancing in public. Anna Halprin, one of the founders of Dance Movement Therapy (DMT), created and facilitated different series of workshops with HIV+ patients as early as 1989 with *Circle the Earth: Dancing with Life on the Line* (1989–1991). These community-led workshops dedicated to HIV+ men and women aimed to "strengthen participants physically, emotionally, mentally, and spiritually" (Halprin).[8] Her work redefined dance as a tool for healing because she tried to mitigate the raw state of illness by distancing movement from aesthetic expectations. The 1980s and 1990s are a time named "non-dance" for that reason. The idea of performing technical prowess seemed futile in a time when illness and death befell the dancer's body.

Since then, scholars and practitioners have explored DMT as an ethnographic method. According to Marlon Bailey: "Performance or performative ethnography is a method of data collection that requires the researcher to actively participate in the very performances and cultural practices that he or she is analyzing. Simply put, for the performance ethnographer, performance is the object and the method of study, as well as the theoretical framework through which the data are analyzed" (2009, 3). DMT allows semiotic activity, discursively conceptualizing dance as speech, message, or expressive communication, fleshing out the narrated event of what dance can concretely do in the social realm. The opening scene of *Good Boy* speaks volumes to the impact of both AZT and healing dance onto Buffard and HIV+ patients more broadly.

> Alone at the back of the stage, Alain Buffard stands still, naked, facing the audience. Hairless, he moves slowly before grabbing an adhesive tape from the floor to tape his penis to his lower abdomen. Hairless and now desexualized, Buffard puts on a pair of tighty-whities, and another one, and another one, creating a massive protective layer.[9]

In her 2017 creative essay *Ce que le sida m'a fait* [*What AIDS Has Done to Me*], Élisabeth Lebovici writes: "Here is an incontinent infant or old man, hips slightly swollen by his textile prosthesis, but still standing" (289). In an interview at the Centre Pompidou in 2021, videographer Philippe Mangeot recalls his sentiment when attending the premiere of *Good Boy* in 1998: "It was a time when the medication made us poop on ourselves. The ones who refused to wear diapers were piling up tighty-whities" (Centre Pompidou). The rawness of both the fecal matter and the vulnerability of the storyteller in first-person narratives reveal the need for individual confession in times of collective battles such as the HIV/AIDS pandemic. This complex relationship to intimacy and the loss of control over one's own excrement is also explored by French author and artist Hervé Guibert who makes a similar confession in his film *La pudeur et l'impudeur* [*Modesty and Shame*] (1992). In one scene, the viewer can see him seated on the toilet with the door left open. It is not by lack of modesty that the door is left ajar but by fear of not being able to open the door himself after having lost the strength and muscle mass to do the most ordinary of activities. In piling up tighty-whities, Buffard similarly stresses and makes public the physical, social, and emotional discomfort he must endure in his intimate life. The piling up routine in this scene exemplifies the type of movement and new mechanisms AIDS created; these mechanisms are usually experienced in the realm of intimacy and are now made public with *Good Boy*.

Traditionally, undergarments are meant to conceal the genitals from the visual and sensorial realms. The act of wearing underwear has become a daily ritual, proof that we are "civilized," that the rawness is cooked, that the individual has accepted social norms. The ritual of piling up tighty-whities is repeated in both *Good For . . .* and *Mauvais genre*. With the multiplication of dancers, the accumulation of tighty-whities forms a new narrative that unifies the group. This collective cohesion creates a type of osmosis while simultaneously shedding light on the standardization of bodies during prophylactic eras. While in *Good Boy* Buffard seems to use this ritual to protect himself from the shame of having to expose bodily secretions and excrement which were effects of his illness, in *Mauvais genre* he hijacks the divide between the proper (civilized) and the improper (raw) by showcasing the forty dancers in the act of piling up underwear in different places: one dancer puts one around his neck to create a collar; others hang them around their waists to form skirts; some form a cluster of panties over their heads and eyes creating headgear that blocks their view; some slip their arms into the leg part of the gear, giving the impression that they are wearing a straitjacket.

This scene seems reminiscent of both Charcot's spectacle of hysterical women and the uncontrollable body of Frau Troffea since both defy social expectations and authorities. The solutions to answer the lack of physical control over female individuals were to criminalize and discipline them. In the context of an epidemic, "individuals become self-regulating subjects" (Green 2008, 176). Regarding the panoptic shadow that watches (or not), that makes itself visible (or not), but forces fear and order, Michel Foucault explains that:

> The historical moment of the disciplines was the moment when an art of the human body was born, which was directed not only at the growth of its skills, nor at the intensification of its subjection, but at the formation of a relation that in the mechanism itself makes it more obedient as it becomes more useful, and conversely . . . Thus discipline produces subjected and practiced bodies, 'docile' bodies. Discipline increases the forces of the body (in economic terms of utility) and diminishes these same forces (in political terms of obedience) . . . They were at work in secondary education at a very early date, later in primary schools; they slowly invested the space of the hospital; and, in a few decades, they restructured the military organization . . . Discipline is a political anatomy of detail. (1975, 137–139)

This sociopolitical perspective has important repercussions on dance since Buffard allows dance to be conceived as a space within which technologies of domination, and techniques of the self contribute to the construction of relationships between body and health. After they put on their tighty-whities, the dancers in *Mauvais Genre* start walking in a circle, one behind the other, in a disciplined rhythm. Order has returned. Their tighty-whities uniform has neutralized their body. The circle reminds us of the classical *corps de ballet* and its harmonious collective that refuses singularity. Yet when the dancers walk in a circle, "c'est moins une communauté indivisée qui apparaît, réconciliée ou non, qu'une multiplication de singularités" ["it is less an undivided community that appears, reconciled or not, than a multiplication of singularities"] (Buffard). Buffard challenges the fantasy of the *corps de ballet* and the illusion of its discipline, privileging the singularities of the bodies decorated by the underwear, each one expressing in their own way their mental and physical state. This scene reveals the necessity to go from a solo piece to an ensemble and from a generational trauma back to individual stories.

> Lying on the ground, his right arm and right leg bent, the dancer moves his shoulder in small convulsions before snapping his elbow on the ground. Same thing on the left: convulsions of the shoulder, elbow banging. Crouching on the floor, arms outstretched under him, head tilted forward, he snaps his forearms together. Body noise. From that position, he leans on his arms and lifts his legs towards the audience. Like a break dancer, he is balanced on his arms, keeping the suspension until he crashes with all his weight on the ground. Body noise.[10]

The body sounds described here refer to medical auscultation, which is traditionally based on the sounds made by the patient's body. In a conventional medical context, the dynamics of auscultation are clear: there is the doctor, that is, an expert who is able to interpret the sound made by the patient, and there is the patient who produces the sound. For Emmanuel Andrès et al.: "In clinical practice, knowing how to distinguish normal and abnormal sounds or noises (vesicular murmur, wheezing, crackling, etc.) remains essential for diagnosis and medical reasoning. Over the past two decades, most of the progress in auscultation has resulted primarily from the development of listening tools, namely the stethoscope itself" (2011, 130). The AIDS epidemic surprised doctors and patients alike as everyone discovered it at the same time. The expertise of the doctor was no longer sufficient for understanding the malady. In this context, Buffard imagines a scene where the individual who makes the sound (the patient) also becomes the expert listener. In *Mauvais genre*, the same auscultation scene occurs, but this time it is with forty dancers. Therefore, it quickly turns into an accumulation of sounds that are impossible to identify. At first, each dancer auscultates their own body as Buffard does in his solo. Then, little by little, duets are formed, and then groups. What's more, multitudes of sounds are made audible with them. From *Good Boy*'s solo to *Mauvais genre*'s group piece, from solitary to group auscultation, it is about showing the transition from an isolating illness to a social pandemic and from self-discipline to collective body policing.

Two years before Buffard's *Good Boy*, French choreographer Boris Charmatz created the ballet *Aatt enen tionon* (1996) in which three dancers (two men and a woman) wore a t-shirt but no underwear, thus revealing their genitalia. Although Charmatz never clearly described this ballet as being about AIDS, it is difficult not to draw links between the title, the date of production, its staging, and the artistic tendency of the time to treat the viral body through a radicalization of the nude. While Buffard made the choice to cover the object of fear and contamination—his penis—Charmatz unveiled it. *Aatt enen tionon* offers a space on three floors, giving the audience three different points of view of the dancers. One can read about Charmatz's piece: "Nudity, paradoxically overexposed by the presence of white T-shirts as the only clothing, questions the viewer about their presence and problematizes their gaze: does nudity overexpose the dancing body or, on the contrary, makes it impossible to read, encrypted by our reading of intimacy, and the hierarchy created by our gaze?" (*Numeridanse.tv*) By hiding or stripping it off, the two choreographers deliberately draw the viewer's eye to the sex of their dancers and force the viewer to ask themselves: Who owns intimacy once it becomes threatening? How can one create privacy in a society that thinks of others as a risk from which it must be protected?

If Buffard did not actively participate in ACT-UP's political efforts and did not consider himself as an activist—contrary to his partner scholar Alain Ménil—he used the stage to create a healing space where it became possible to reclaim a lost intimacy. His triptych is testament to a time where dancing was an act of resistance, and viral dance was challenging the very definition of dance as an aesthetic and athletic art. Today, with the COVID-19 pandemic, similar patterns of marginalization occur, and a similar need to use dance as a way to resist forced immobility also emerged.

COVID-19: MOVING AGAINST SOCIAL DISTANCING

In March 2020, Ohioan Keara Wilson a.k.a "Queen Keke" posted on her TikTok account a video shot in her bedroom, in which she performs a dance she created to the sound of Megan Thee Stallion's *Savage*.

> Facing the camera, Queen Keke sticks her tongue out while smiling: "I'm a savage," her hands clap. To the lyrics "Classy, bougie, ratchet," she places her right hand on the back of her head, left hand down, her hip kicks up sideway. "Sassy, moody, nasty," her body parallel to the camera, she arches her back, "Acting stupid," her two hands around her head, fingers stretched out, thumbs touching her temples: "What's happening? Bitch / I'm a savage."

No lighting, no scenography, no costume. Only a bedroom, Queen Keke, and her phone. The video went viral and became the most played on the app for that month, accumulating more than 7.5 billion views. This viral dance is symptomatic of a moment, as in March 2020, the COVID-19 pandemic forced global lockdowns in order to slow the spread of SARS-CoV-2. Consequently, venues and dance studios closed worldwide. For months, the only places remaining to move were one's own house, outdoor or rural spaces, and the internet. Social media application TikTok became one of the spaces where movers reimagined their relationship to space, traditional geographies of dance and rethought the need of aesthetization. Created by Chinese group ByteDance, TikTok saw a phenomenal rise in users and cultural visibility during the first lockdown. As of August 2020, the app was downloaded more than eighty million times in the United States alone and reached two billion downloads worldwide. Social media and digital technologies value the idea of "going viral," as a post, a video, a comment is valued by the number of likes it receives, by the number of times it is retweeted. Therefore, when a dance goes viral, the reach of its movements and influence is immense, redefining the very idea of border and geography. "Infectious dances," as *The New York Times* names them, or viral dances such as Queen Keke's, form a global language that instills global values, views, and foreign aesthetics, entering domestic spaces and transforming local aesthetics.

Since the end of the 1970s and the development of the first digital viruses, the viral metaphor goes far beyond the medical to find itself in other spheres like technology, politics, and media. The terms used to talk about a digital virus are the same as those used to talk about a biological virus: propagation, host cell, infection, hygiene and computer virology, etc. Here, medical terms have colonized the digital sphere through new semantics. Thanks to an already-established virtual life, the rise of digital socialization and education during the 21st century has prepared the world to culturally manage the COVID-19 pandemic.

However, the geography of dance only changed for those used to frequenting institutional spaces or traditional dance studios. In France, dance is still recognized by the places where it is made visible. The street, the Internet, or one's home are spaces historically occupied by minorities. A club or a Maison des Jeunes et de la Culture [Youth and Culture Center] are not institutionalized places of culture dissemination since, firstly, they are not subsidized by the State, being outside the approved stages; second, streets and clubs welcome bodies that belong to colonial imaginaries which have created what is acceptable to be shown on stage to the dominant audience. Dance follows a well-established geographic and economic order: white dancers belong to the stage, to the Republic, while dancers of color belong to the club, the *banlieue*, and the street. The latter are unsophisticated, raw spaces where traditional scenography with lighting, costume or mise-en-scène are replaced by a standing crowd and concrete floor, or a bedroom as in the case of Queen Keke. Acknowledging that we live in a time where the domestic is constantly "contaminated" by the global and vice versa, where the virtual injects global images in local spaces, shows how COVID-19 challenges this historical divide between spaces of creation.

During the first lockdown of the COVID-19 pandemic in March 2020, other viral, social phenomenon occurred, such as the rise of anti-Asian hate. Black Lives Matter protests also went global after the death of George Floyd and an ongoing epidemic of political brutality. Anti-immigrant hate speech flourished and called for heightened border restrictions and control. Using the health crisis as an excuse to legitimize the closure of borders, far-right French group Génération Identitaire went to the Spanish border in January 2021 with the intention to prevent any migrant from entering France. Founded in 2012, the organization was dissolved shortly after this last event, having officially been recognized as a white supremacist, Islamophobic, and neo-fascist organization. Nevertheless, it is important to understand how they are merely the product of structural violence set up in neocolonial contexts which promote regionalism for the sake of purity. The repetition of hateful patterns fuels stigma experience. Whether it was Saint Vitus' dancers criminalized by townships for disrupting local life, HIV+ individuals blamed for their sexual behaviors, or Asian communities accused of exporting COVID-19, stigmatization remains part of pandemic narratives. As an engaged dance scholar, I decided to respond to this hostile environment by offering dance workshops to immigrant people, a marginalized population often forgotten in times of national and global crisis, settling in the south of France.

> Right hand covers her eyes. Left hand covers her mouth. Right hand's index finger covers her mouth, as the left hand comes down. While stretching her arm, the index finger moves away from her mouth, in front of her. She holds her finger in the air as her head turns around trying to look behind her.[11]

This movement was created by Rhizlane, a woman from Morocco who participated in the dance workshops I offered in Saint Gaudens, France, from February to June 2021, as part of my ongoing practice-based research project called On Board(hers).[12] I created this series of contemporary dance workshops and performances in 2018 in Ohio, in the United States, in order to respond to an urgent social and psychological neglect of the so-called contemporary migration "crisis." Offered exclusively to immigrants, On Board(hers) deploys a trauma-informed technique using movement, language, and affect theory. It models best practices for transformational community engagement through storytelling, while showing the functions of intellectual creativity and the importance of activism at a scholarly level. The methodology used in On Board(hers) is inscribed in the field of DMT and inspired by Halprin's healing dance. It is destined to people with no particular dance training who have not been shaped by one particular technique. This level of physical rawness allows the participants to develop a more authentic relationship to their body and their story.

Since 2020 and the COVID-19 pandemic, physical contact is prohibited, sanitary measures are imposed, and borders are becoming more policed. These measures are a clear reminder of how the AIDS crisis was used as an excuse to further control spaces and practices belonging to the margin. Governments tried different measures which led to the criminalization of marginalized groups: closing queer spaces, encouraging the outing of serological status in the workplace, creating the "4 Hs myth" (Homosexuals, Heroin-users, Hemophiliacs, and Haitians) in order to create a narrative based on shame and stigma. The COVID-19 pandemic revealed pre-existing social distancing of minority groups and senior citizens, inequalities in the face of access to digital technologies and education, and the rise of domestic violence which almost doubled during the different lockdowns. Of the 22 women I worked with in France, 18 came from a local shelter for women victims of domestic abuse. The population I worked with did not have access to high-speed internet[13] or a domestic space that could welcome such a practice. Therefore, we met in-person with masks on and using social distancing. In the middle of the pandemic, these workshops were, for some, the only human contact they had during their week.

Rhizlane's movement is symptomatic of a larger discussion on viral dance and the impact of pandemics on immigrants' rights to move. Covering her eyes and her mouth with her own hands and silencing herself with her own finger show the mechanisms immigrants had to develop in order to navigate their new life in the host country. During our workshops, participants put into motion the different levels of isolation they encountered, the ways in which the pandemic accentuated their invisibilization within the space they occupy, and their vulnerability. The type of movements they created were mostly about the violence of the media toward immigrants and the impossibility to meet or interact with locals. Like the WE-Program mentioned in the introduction and the applications mostly focusing on solo creations in times of isolation, the movements created by the On Board(hers) participants were either a direct response to COVID-19 or represented the impact of social, emotional, cultural, and linguistic distancing onto their life, such as Rhizlane's movement. It also made evident that concepts such as "social distancing" and "new geographies of dance" are only new to those whose access to spaces and social activities are never endangered. The consequences of isolation are greater for immigrants than for local citizens. Without proof of integration into the French society, undocumented immigrants are denied access to a temporary visa or permanent residency. Two of the participants I worked with over these five months were deported because they were not able to find a job or show their social integration into local life.

At first, the goal of On Board(hers) was to create a sense of belonging for immigrant women settled in the United States and to develop personal narratives that would counter anti-immigration discourses of the Trump administration. The COVID-19 pandemic added new needs and layers of discrimination to immigrant communities. In 2021, in France, On Board(hers) became a way for the participants to escape anonymity by reclaiming their right to move and be visible in the city. The performance we offered in June 2021 meant to highlight the participants' journeys and force empathy. Toward the end of the performance, participants taught their movements to the audience. This moment of movement exchange between locals and immigrants is in line with the ways in which global gestures on TikTok contaminate domestic spaces. By learning On Board(hers) dancers' movements, local audience members accepted stories that did not belong to them and gestures that did not reflect their own journey. Exploring vulnerability, emotions, and bodies as raw materials makes possible a response and a counter-discourse to official narratives.

CONCLUSION

The examples in this chapter seek out a raw aesthetic in order to return to an undisciplined form of movement and challenge a classical vision of the dancing body as non-human. Here, the desire to dance well, to achieve perfection through technical prowess is replaced by the dancers' need to rebel. Rawness exposes underlying violence: as she sweats and foams among hundreds of other dancers in trance, Frau Troffea refuses the gender propriety imposed by her time; when Alain Buffard tapes his penis on his lower abdomen, he reveals the castrating consequences of shame and stigma rhetoric; Queen Keke and other viral TikTok Tok dancers are symptomatic of a moment in history which combines several epidemics of violence and social revolts; the self-silencing movement created by Rhizlane speaks volumes to the targeting of marginalized groups in times of global health crisis. From a Medical Humanities perspective, it seems impossible to isolate epidemics from one another. On the contrary, acknowledging their porosity sheds light on recurring phenomena and, one could hope, an opportunity to learn from them.

BIBLIOGRAPHY

Abrahams, Andrew (dir.) and Anna Halprin. 2010. *Positive Motion: Challenging AIDS through Dance and Ritual.* Documentary, The USC Center for Visual Anthropology, USA.

Autour du film "*Good Boy, histoire d'un solo.*" Rencontre avec Philippe Mangeot et Marie-Hélène Rebois: Interview, Centre Pompidou: Paris.

Bailey, Marlon. 2009. "Performance as Intravention: Ballroom Culture and the Politics of HIV/AIDS in Detroit" in *Souls. A Critical Journal of Black Politics, Culture, and Society*: Chicago: University of Illinois, Vol. 11. 3.

Bonthius, Daniel O. and Bahri Karacay. 2003. "Sydenham's Chorea: Not Gone and Not Forgotten" in *Seminars in Pediatric Neurology*, Vol. 110, No. 1 (March).
Buffard, Alain. 1998. *Good Boy*: Paris.
———. 2002. *Good For . . .* Paris.
———. 2003. *Mauvais Genre*: Paris.
———. 2005. *My Lunch with Anna*. Film, France: PI:ES Production.
Campbell, Alyson and Dirk Gindt, eds. 2018. *Viral Dramaturgies: HIV and AIDS in Performance in the Twenty-First Century*: London: Palgrave Macmillan.
Charmatz, Boris. 1996. *Aatt enen tionon*. La Halle aux Grains-Scène nationale de Blois.
Colette-Folliot, Valérie. 2015. *L'Apesanteur Dansée Ou le Corps Dansant Glorieux: une Idée, un Concept, une Réalité - Tome I*: Gelos: Echappée Belle.
Daniel O. Bonthius and Bahri Karacay. 2003. "Sydenham's Chorea: Not Gone and Not Forgotten" in *Seminars in Pediatric Neurology*, Vo110, No 1 (March): 11–19.
Emmanuel, Andrès, Christian Brandt and Mustapha Mecili. 2011. "Progrès et innovation dans le domaine de l'auscultation" in *Pédagogie*: John Libbey Eurotext, 17 (2).
Foucault, Michel (1975). *Discipline and Punish. The Birth of the Prison*: Translated by Alan Sheridan. New York: Random House.
———. 2003. *Le pouvoir psychiatrique, Cours au Collège de France. 1973–1974*.
Frimat, Francois. 2011. *Qu'est-ce que la danse contemporaine?* Paris: PUF.
Green, Jill. 2008. "Ethiques et politiques de la santé en éducation de la danse aux Etats-Unis" in Sylvie Fortin, dir. *Danse et santé. Du corps intime au corps social*: Quebec: Presses de l'Université du Québec.
Guibert, Hervé. 1992. *La pudeur et l'impudeur*. Documentary, France: BQHL Productions.
Halprin, Anna. 1990. *Carry Me Home:* USA.
Hecker, Justus. 1885. *The Dancing Mania of the Middle Ages*. Trans. By G.B. Babington. New York: Humboldt Publishing Company. Online access.
Hecker, Justus. 1835. *The Epidemics of the Middle Ages*. Trans. by G.B. Babington. Online access.
Johnson, Brian D. 2019. "How a Typo Created a Scapegoat for the AIDS Epidemic" in *Maclean's*: online post, April 17.
Kabir, Ananya Jahanara. 2021. "From the Black Death to Black Dance: Choreomania as Cultural Symptom" in *Cambridge Journal of Postcolonial Literary Inquiry*: Stanford University, 8(2), 270–276.
Lebovici, Élisabeth. 2017. *Ce que le sida m'a fait*. Dijon: Les Presses du Réel.
Marineli, Filio et al. 2013. "Mary Mallon (1869–1938) and the history of typhoid fever." *Annals of gastroenterology*. Vol. 26, 2: 132–134.
McKay, Richard A. 2017. *Patient Zero and the Making of the AIDS Epidemic*. Chicago & London: The University of Chicago Press.
Megan Thee Stallion. 2020. *Savage*. Music, 300 Entertainment Label, USA.
Perreault, Marie□Anne. 2020. "Freud, Foucault et les hystériques: Résistance contre le pouvoir psychiatrique" in *Ithaque* 27, 47–66.
Queen Keke. 2020. *Savage*. Dance video, TikTok, USA.

Rebois, Marie-Hélène, dir. 2020. *Good Boy, histoire d'un solo*. Documentary, France: Daphnie Productions.
Routy, Jean-Pierre. 2011. *Ce que le sida a changé*. Montreal: Héliotrope.
Schechter, DC. 1975. *St Vitus' dance and rheumatic disease:* New York State Journal of Medicine 75, 1091–1102.
Stephenson, Barry. 2001. "Charcot's Theater of Hysteria." *Journal of Ritual Studies* 15, no. 1: 27–37.
Waller, John. 2009. *The Dancing Plague. The Strange, True Story of an Extraordinary Illness*. Vienna: Sourcesbooks.

NOTES

1. See *Playing for Life. Performance in Africa in the Age of AIDS* by Louise Manon Bourgault (2003); *How to Make Dances in an Epidemic: Tracking Choreography in the Age of AIDS* by David Gere (2004); *Ce que le sida m'a fait* by Élisabeth Lebovici (2017); *Viral Dramaturgies: HIV and AIDS in Performance in the Twenty-First Century* edited by Alyson Campbell and Dirk (2018).
2. https://www.we-program.com.
3. See Valérie Colette-Folliot. 2015.
4. Such as, among others: *Kleinlawel, Strassburgische Chronik, der kurtze Beschreibung von Ankunfft, Erbaw, und Erweiterung der Statt Strassburg, wie auch vom Leben, Regierung, und Absterben der Bischoffen daselbsten* (1625); or *Bulletin de la Société pour la Conservation des Monuments Historiques d'Alsace.*
5. Indeed, the status of Gaétan Dugas as patient zero was a myth. As part of a 1984 study, Dugas "was renamed Patient O, with the letter 'O' standing for 'Out-of-California.' Somewhere along the paper trail, the 'O' got confused with a zero" (Johnson 2019).
6. See Richard A. McKay. 2017.
7. For the purpose of this article, I will include my own descriptions of the performances.
8. From Anna Halpring's website https://www.annahalprin.org.
9. My description.
10. My description.
11. My description.
12. www.onboardhers.com.
13. Parallel to my work in France, On Board(hers) also facilited groups in Mexico (led by Gloria Flores) and Germany (led by Flor Turiace). For both of them, the internet became one major platform to recruit new participants, and dance safely in 2021.

Chapter Seven

State of Sexual Exception

SARS-CoV-2, HIV, and Sexual Citizenship in Pandemic Times

CJ Gomolka

Since the emergence of SARS-CoV-2 at the end of December 2019 in Wuhan, China, information about the coronavirus has proliferated through a rhizomatic network of discourses dominating international airwaves and penetrating practically the entirety of lived experience across the globe. Given the similar epidemiological and epistemological terrain that they seem to share, it may not be all that surprising that the specter of the AIDS crisis was redeployed within the mediatized discursive grid that attempted to bring some type of intelligibility to the SARS-CoV-2 pandemic and its global effects. From mid-March 2020, journalists, politicians, doctors, sociopolitical organizations, and associations in France wrote into the media circuit epidemiological comparisons and etiological theories comparing HIV and SARS-CoV-2, mobilized queer sociosexual practices, and pulled from S/M sartorial play in conversations about risk reduction during pandemic-time sex.

This chapter will analyze the epistemological effects of this informational expanse on conceptualizations of sex, illness, and sexual citizenship in France through what I am calling a state of sexual exception since the start of the SARS-CoV-2 pandemic. This state of sexual exception was nourished at least in part by the seemingly extraordinary pandemic proscription of corporeal proximity and produced, what I will argue was, the subsequent recasting of the contours of sexual citizenship models through provisional appeals to the more fluid conceptualizations of queer sociosexual practice and identity. As I will show, this contingent remodeling of modalities of sexual citizenship in France was operationalized against the media backdrop of appropriated HIV/

AIDS discourses, mythologies, and histories used as epistemological reference points, however erroneous, for the desultory national and individual orientations to the emergent SARS-CoV-2 virus. This newly invested mediatic proximity between conceptualizations of HIV/AIDS and SARS-CoV-2 cultivated an epistemological circuit between sex, illness, individual, and nation used to provide often crude justifications for state "safety" protocols while simultaneously fostering the reconceptualization of sexual citizenship models for pandemic times. Finally, these appeals to sexual exception led to the emergence of novel biotech sexual solidarity models and queer techno-kinships even as they often invisibilized the important risk-reduction strategies of the HIV/AIDS discourses they mobilized and (re)stigmatized those queer individuals and collectivities that wield them.

STATE OF SEXUAL EXCEPTION IN BIOTECH TIMES

The global proliferation of SARS-CoV-2 ushered in what might be termed a state of sexual exception, that is, a regulatory epistemological and biotech regime that both produced and was justified by pandemic-time protocols for body proximity and that put pressure on national and individual conceptualizations of sex, sexual possibility, and sexual citizenship in France during times of health crisis. Indeed, the global flow of SARS-CoV-2 and the attendant state-mandated preliminary lockdown measures intended to stem its tide ripped many of us from intimate and social engagement thus threatening one of our most cherished of human impulses: the gravitational and libidinal pull of body proximity. As an end to lockdown and return to a sense of normalcy became embroiled in the rising case numbers and attendant deaths, digitized almost to the moment by the necrotech infographics of governmental and news agencies, time lost its predictable cadence, ebbing and flowing more noticeably to the baleful whims of Western biopolitics. By mid-March, the global flow of SARS-CoV-2 had collided with the formidable and rapacious machine of Western extractivist capitalism, grinding its gears to a veritable halt and exposing cavernous inequities plaguing certain global and local minoritized populations.[1]

Even with the almost complete and utter collapse of most Western state and economic systems, sex, or the possible lack thereof, seemed to occupy a primordial, and perhaps overly dramatized, mediatized positioning in France in relation to the global effects of SARS-CoV-2. Leveraging clickbait algorithms to attract anxious *internautes* [internet users] with titles like "Pour se protéger du covid, les autorités canadiennes conseillent le 'glory hole'" ["To protect against covid, Canadian authorities recommend 'glory holes'"][2], "Un lien entre Covid-19 et VIH?" ["A link between Covid-19 and HIV?"], and

"Coronavirus: la sexualité confinée" ["Coronavirus: sexuality under lockdown"], mainstream media outlets and social media platforms across France[3] rushed to imagine putatively novel corporeal epistemologies and praxes that centered our individual and collective need to get off while simultaneously exposing biopolitical anxieties concerning the body's relation to stasis, space, desire, illness, disease, death, protection, proximity, time, and community. Folded within these epistemologies and practices were contingent formulations of sexual citizenships and sexual subjectivities as well as exceptional (and exceptions to) sexual practices, temporarily sanctioned and naturalized through the regulatory biopolitical and biotech scripts mapping the terrain of possible sexual exploits during pandemic times, what I have elsewhere called "biotechsex" (Gomolka 2021).[4]

Giorgio Agamben (2005) understood the "state of exception," and the exceptional measures enacted in its name, as existing in a paradoxical relationship with politics and law, indeed, existing at their limits (1). For Agamben, "[t]he state of exception is neither external nor internal to the juridical order, and the problem of defining it concerns precisely a threshold, or a zone of indifference, where inside and outside do not exclude each other but rather blur with each other" (23). Similarly, he explains, individual subjects or collective populations can be subjected to the effects of this obfuscating threshold, altering, confusing, or eradicating their subjectivity, giving the state of exception a productive and definitional role in the management of life technologies as well as the (de)optimization of life and therefore an exceptionally biopolitical dimension (3).[5] Jasbir Puar (2007) expands on the linguistic play of the exceptional nature of the exception contending that "[e]xceptionalism paradoxically signals distinction from (to be unlike, dissimilar) as well as excellence (imminence, superiority), suggesting a departure from yet mastery of linear teleologies of progress" (3). In this way, we might interrogate which distinct sexual practices, discourses, and identities were called into the public arena for manipulation and mobilization since the start of the pandemic in order to "rescue" sexual subjects from the seemingly exceptional position of sexless lives. Similarly, we might identify which exceptional and exceptions to dominant modes of sexual citizenships were rendered operational in France at this time and to what ends.

By state of sexual exception during COVID times then, I do not mean a state with no sex. The semio-epistemological play inherent in exception and exceptionalism points rather to a state in which, because of the suspension of normal state functioning, sex was made to manifest through exception and in exceptional ways. Indeed, so that the narratives and scripts of sexual exception might gain purchase as they were produced and sanctioned through appeals to national health, safety, and security in the public sphere, the imagined community of "normal" sexual actors and activities needed to be reconceived through less rigid and austere sexual lexicons and epistemologies suggesting sexual citizenship as necessarily tensile in seemingly sexo-calimatous circumstances.[6] As the next section will show, iterative national and mediatized discourses on sex effected this reconceptualization through the proliferation of an array of queer subjectivities and practices into the public sphere. Insofar as this shift in sexual citizenship models relied on the larger media apparatus for transmission, it should also be understood as part of the biotech circuits of technocapitalism and what Paul Preciado (2013) has called the pharmacopornographic regime (33).[7] Of course, mobilizing queer subjectivities and practices does not mean that normalized and dominant modalities of sexuality, sexual practices, and sexual citizenships were excluded from this mediatized matrix of discursive production on sex during the pandemic. Rather, an understanding of the functioning of the state of sexual exception must take into consideration the dynamic interplay and negotiations between epistemological and biopolitical modalities of existent and emergent sexualities, sexual subjectivities, sexual practices, and sexual histories. To this end, the next section will analyze some of the mediatized state of sexual exception protocols proposed to sexual actors during the SARS-CoV-2 pandemic. In order to better understand their sociopolitical and cultural impact, these protocols need to be situated within larger epistemological circuits that form and inform our understandings of disease, sex, individual, and nation. Finally, this next section will suggest that these state of sexual exception protocols were not only active in effecting reconceptualizations of "normal" sexual citizenship in France during the pandemic. They were also ultimately productive of novel biotech sexual solidarities and queer techno-kinship models that might be mobilized outside of pandemic times in order to enhance queer and non-queer minority networks (trans)locally and (trans)nationally.

QUEER SEX PROTOCOLS, BIOTECH SEXUAL SOLIDARITY, QUEER TECHNO-KINSHIPS

I would like to start with a series of headlines that address sexuality during the COVID-19 pandemic:

> Comment bien vivre sa sexualité sans propager le Covid 19
> (How to best live your sexuality without spreading Covid 19)
>
> —vih.org, 2020

Un masque pour séduire son partenaire?
(Masking up to seduce your partner?)

—*Courrier-Picard*, 2020

Make it a little kinky.

—NYC Health, 2020

Use barriers, like walls (e.g., glory holes), that allow for sexual contact but prevent close face-to-face contact.

—British Colombia Center for Disease Control, 2020

In mid-March 2020, Thomas Seymat (2020), digital journalist and professor of journalism at Sciences Po Lyon, framed desire in the age of SARS-CoV-2 within a lexicon of temptation, loss, and protection romanticized through the biotech aesthetics of the lead images of his *EuroNews* article, "Sexe, drague et coronavirus: comment se protéger à l'heure de Covid-19," ["Sex, Dating, and Coronavirus: How to Keep Safe in Covid Times"]. The images insist on the global nature of the crisis, two young couples' "final" embrace in March 2020 at the Milan and Rio de Janeiro train stations, even as the language of the article anchors in France the raw anxiety of affective proximity alluded to by the title. The almost apocalyptic sentiment of the images is biomedically enhanced through the by-now iconic sartorial accessorizing of pandemic-time *tenue* [dress]: surgical blue masks and protective gloves (PPE) highlighting the new biotech frontier, what Paul Preciado has called "le préservatif social des masses" ["social condoms for the masses"] (2020b), between desire, bodies, and disease. The bulk of the article itself is slightly less dramatic providing embryonic developments on viral transmission and possible risk-reduction protocols based on New York city's "safe sex and Covid-19" guide. Perhaps unable to resist the lure of false equivalencies, Seymat entreats the need for these protocols through a hypertextual analogy that also seems to serve as a portent: an embedded link to a May 29, 2014, *NewYork* article by Tim Murphy entitled "7 New Yorkers Remember the Early Days of the AIDS Epidemic" that doubles as a reminder of the number of AIDS-related deaths from 1981–1994 in New York.[8] Maïa Mazaurette opens her opinion piece on sex and the pandemic for *Le Monde* in May by decrying the loss of the habitually sweaty salaciousness of the summer months chilled down by, what she calls, the twin pillars of pandemic seduction technique: "transparency" and "prudency" (2020). Referencing a state of sexual exception indexed through an assemblage of spatial, affective, temporal, and historical intensities that point to lost time, bodies, and desires, she states: "Pandémie oblige, les aventures érotiques sont reportées à des jours meilleurs et la spontanéité en prend un coup . . . Toutes proportions gardées, nous voici revenus aux angoisses des années sida, quand certains refusaient même de serrer des mains" ["Pandemic necessity: erotic adventures put off until better days and as a result spontaneity suffers . . . Relatively speaking, here we are back to the anxieties of the AIDS years, when some even refused to shake hands"] (2020). If Mazaurette laments the ostensible loss of pre-pandemic physical proximity through reckless rearticulations of mythologies concerning HIV transmission, others registered anxieties concerning illness and sex for the future, specifically the end-of-lockdown period (11 May—15 June) in France. According to a late-July, auto-administered study of 3,018 hexagonal French individuals conducted by Ifop (*Institut français d'opinion publique*) for the site PornHub, sex for singles from the beginning of the pandemic through post-lockdown has been especially difficult: sexual liberty constrained by disciplinary pandemic protocols that circumscribe sex within a biopolitics inflected by austerity, anxiety, and stigmatizing trauma. Indeed, François Kraus, director of the Gender, Sexualities, and Sexual Health Center at Ifop, states: "La Covid-19 constitue un frein à la liberté sexuelle des célibataires . . . en tant que source de contrainte et de crainte, en particulier envers les personnes travaillant dans des secteurs exposés au virus . . . qui n'est pas sans rappeler la stigmatization des maladies du VIH dans les 'années SIDA'" ["Covid-19 represents an obstacle to sexual freedom for singles . . . as a source of constraint and fear, in particular toward those working in sectors exposed to the virus . . . reminding us of the stigmatization of those living with HIV during the 'AIDS years'"] (Col 2020).[9] While the next section of this article will interrogate the specific logics that subtend the technoterrain of mediatized coverage that brought HIV/AIDS and SARS-CoV-2 into interesting relations of proximity and (un)willed adjacency,[10] for the moment I would like to tarry a bit in the biotech economies of sexual anxiety, trauma, and sexual exception(alism) produced during the first several months of the pandemic and linked more generally to the ways in which HIV and SARS-CoV-2 were made to co-exist in global media during this time.

The headlines that open this section suggest that exceptional sex advice and sex-based protocols for the generalized population of sexual actors during the pandemic turned a little queer. Through appeals to exceptional practices and sexual expediency—the S/M-esque aestheticization of face coverings as seduction technique during sex, kink phantasm, and the cruising and erotic architectures of glory holes—state sexual protocols in COVID times reimagined the contours of normative sexual citizenship as less rigidly puritan by folding raw quirk and play into an otherwise rather bland list of risk-reduction measures for sexual actors. Moreover, the idea of a state of sexual exception allowed national discourse to summon certain non-normative sexual practices and discourses from the unnerving hinterlands of conventionally undesirable sexual praxis in order to satisfy the needs of sexual citizens newly confronted with an ostensibly state-imposed onanistic or erotico-digitized sexual existence.

As the lockdown began in mid-March 2020, French online media outlets quickly loaded the body into varied biotech circuits of sexual activity and virtual-communal erotic experiences thus mapping out a cartography of novel sexual subjectivities and citizenships that might be called upon in these seemingly exceptional sexual circumstances. Indeed, some media outlets exposed, not without some cheek, the ins-and-outs of gloryhole protocols (Duranton 2020; Durin-Valois 2020; Giard 2020), the use of virtually connected sex toys (Durin-Valois 2020; Sikouk 2020), the reconceptualization of (virtual) "5 à 7" ["workplace quickies"] ("L'activité sexuelle des Français" 2020), and the liberatory psycho-physiological experiences of virtual sex, broadly defined (Viala 2021). Others registered moves toward (non-or remunerated) individualized, erotic virtual experiences (Giami 2021, 6), imagined the pandemic as a way to loosen the sociocultural constraints on Western monogamic practices (*Sexe et amours confinés* 2020), or proposed the erotization of lockdown itself through participation in "Erosticonfinement" ["desire-during-lockdown"], a biotech offshoot of the artistic and political project *Erosticratie* that proposed erotic videos and readings from individual users throughout the lockdown on Skype and their YouTube channel (*Erosticratie* 2020).[11]

Of course, very few of these sexual experiences and practices are new per se. It is rather their incorporation into mainstream public discourse on possible modalities of sexual citizenship through appeals to a state of sexual exception during the pandemic that makes them novel in any way. The framing of these experiences and practices as exceptions to and exceptional normative sexual practice(s), often visually through media titles that emphasize the contingent and mutually constitutive nature of exceptional sexual practices and pandemic protocols,[12] was important in order to avoid any overly egregious deviation from the heteropatriarchal topography of idealized (hetero)sexual citizenship models existent in France (Provencher 2007, 7–28). Appealing to these exceptional practices in this way also situated them tightly within the coextensive field of self-serving narratives of French exceptionalism and exception that attempted to index all pandemic-time individual and national public policy within the more generalized landscape of state of exception lexicons and contemporary biopolitical discourse. Indeed, on 16 March 2020, while discussing state lockdown and pandemic protocols French President Emmanuel Macron announced: "Jamais la France n'avait dû prendre de telles décisions, évidemment exceptionnelles . . . Mais croyez-moi, cet effort que je vous demande, je sais qu'il est inédit, mais les circonstances nous obligent" ["Never before has France needed to make such decisions, evidently exceptional . . . But believe me, what I'm asking of you (French citizens), I know that it's unprecedented, but the current circumstances make this necessary"] (Macron 2020).[13]

While the aforementioned media productions are only a small cross section of the constellation of mediatized discourses on sex and the pandemic since mid-March 2020,[14] they are illustrative of more generalized efforts to frame pandemic times through discourses frontloaded by anxiety, loss, exception, and trauma often extrapolated from the individual to the national. In his March address to the French nation, Macron (2020) invoked the state of exception in a bellicose tone, urging calm, pointing to the inevitable social, societal, and cultural losses of the pandemic, calling on individual citizens to rethink [*innover*] social and interpersonal bonds within the delimited bounds of physical distancing protocols, while repeatedly pointing to the need for a "sens des responsabilités et de la solidarité" ["sense of responsibility and solidarity"]. Through the invocation, no less than six times, of the phrase "nous sommes en guerre" ["we are at war"] and the mix of individualist and universalist rhetoric, "[h]issons-nous individuellement et collectivement à la hauteur du moment . . . [j]e sais, mes chers compatriots, pouvoir compter sur vous" ["let's rise, individually and collectively, to the moment . . . I know, my fellow countrymen, that I can count on you"] (Macron 2020), the dynamic circuit between trauma, anxiety, loss, and national and individual safety and security was channeled through the neoliberal notion of individual responsibility to the nation linking thus biopolitics and universalism through the Latin *communitas—cum* (with) and *munus* (duty, tax, tribute, gift). To be sure, this exceptional discursive framing is rather ironic given France's well-established, truculent stance against communitarian discourse.

Of course, as many theorists have shown, one's duties to the nation are always already sexualized within the hetero-capitalist, imperialist structures of Western sexual citizenship models (Bell and Binnie 2000, 10; Provencher 2007, 7–28). Perhaps then it is not all that surprising to see queer sexual protocols rendered novel and operational, if exceptional, modalities of sexual citizenship in many mainstream media circuits during the pandemic. Indeed, as the previously mentioned media discourses attest, the anxiety and trauma provoked by the possibility of a generalized state of sexual exception, one that might have deprived sexual actors of intimate sociality, the state of future sexual citizens, and therefore fragilize the biopolitical integrity of the state, was by mid-March already circulating within the collective nationalized imaginary and response to the pandemic. A year out, these anxieties are being fleshed out in studies outlining biopolitical concerns over declining birthrates (de Charette 2021; Leclair 2021; Valo 2021) as well as lower life expectancy and drops in marriages (Papon and Beaumel 2021) all of which are linked to the physio-psychological effects of the virus thus highlighting a dynamic and mutually constitutive circuit between illness, sex, the individual, and the state. As viable and effective preemptive technologies against SARS-CoV-2 emerged early in 2021, the interpretative grid expressing the relationality between conceptual elements within this circuit has shifted from anxieties concerning individual and national hyposexual disruption to the commercialization of appeals to both individual and national libidinal compulsions. The vaccination campaigns for the *Agence régionale de santé Provence-Alpes Côte d'Azur* [Regional Health Agency Provence-Alpes Côte d'Azur] are a provocative example of biopolitical appeals to raw desire: a series of seductive images of (sexual) life "after Covid" (read: after vaccination) including a particularly suggestive fluid-swapping session between the mouths of two men with the tagline, "Oui, le vaccin peut avoir des effets désirables. A chaque vaccination c'est la vie qui reprend. Vaccinons-nous." ["Yes, the vaccine can have desirable effects. With each vaccination, life starts back up. Let's get vaccinated"].

However, access to this digitized cartography of novel erotic experiences operationalized during COVID times, and therefore participation in this constitutive citizenship circuit, was inequitably distributed across racialized, gender, and class lines. Indeed, many of those designated pandemic "frontline workers" were women of color and immigrant populations from extra-muros Paris (Vallaud-Belkacem and Laugier 2020) who, because of endemic pre-pandemic, socio-economic inequalities and the psycho-physiological stress of being considered momentarily "essential" (Diallo 2020), were less likely flush with the time and economics necessary to participate in the leisurely exploration of proposed sexual protocols. Additionally, as Pierre Manière (2018) has shown, many of these same minoritized populations reside in areas affected by a "fracture numérique" ["digital divide"], lacking the highspeed internet access (physical and financial) needed to fully participate in or even know about these digitized circuits of (trans)national eroticism.[15]

We might then modify Ann Cvetkovich's (2003) language and consider the SARS-CoV-2 crisis as productive of a "national sexual trauma" figuring among other "nation-and world-defining events" like AIDS, the Holocaust, and the Great Wars (125). Cvetkovich states: "[t]rauma makes itself felt in everyday practices and nowhere more insidiously or insistently than in converting what was once pleasure into the specter of loss or in preventing the acknowledgment of such losses. It may be a necessity rather than a luxury to consider trauma's impact on sexual life or how its effects are mediated through forms of oppression such as homophobia" (127). Indeed, many national, queer, and not-for-profit media outlets and associations including *Komitid*, *Têtu*, *The Conversation,* and AIDES attested to an increase in LGBTQphobia during the SARS-CoV-2 crisis resurrecting, or perhaps just re-exposing, the biopolitical circuit between sex, sexuality, trauma, and disease linked historically and epistemologically in the West to HIV/AIDS (Beaucamp 2020; Brancourt 2020; Crimp 1989; Ljungcrantz and Gustavson 2020; Pézeril 2020). It is without a doubt essential to avoid overly facile analogical analyses between the AIDS crisis and the SARS-CoV-2 pandemic. However, it is equally vital to expose any bio/necropolitical overlap in failed or exclusionary sociopolitical policies or discriminatory discourses concerning LGBTQ populations between the two. This will be especially important in order to interrogate the continued operational failures of certain state policies concerning LGBTQ populations as well as to illustrate how difficult it can be to disengage phobic health policy and discrimination economies. As such, we might consider especially salient the necropolitical, exclusionary housing policies for at-risk LGBTQ youth (Tanguy 2020), the thanato-theological, international analogies between SARS-CoV-2, homosexuality, and divine punishment mediatized in France through the magazine *Têtu* (Rauglaudre 2020), as well as the generalized stigmatization of LGBTQ populations during the SARS-CoV-2 crisis that affected access to medical care and psycho-physiological health resources, created precarious living and work situations, and heightened exposure to physical violence all placing LGBTQ individuals at higher risk of contracting SARS-CoV-2 (Dunbar 2020; "Urgences LGBTQI" 2020).

For some queer activists, the specific trauma of having lived through the AIDS crisis "rend plus outillé à identifier les invariants (éléments qui restent constants) des épidémies et à développer des ressources sans attendre des réactions des pouvoirs publics et concrètes" [makes one better equipped to identify the invariants (elements that remain constant) of epidemics and to develop resources without waiting for concrete reactions from public authorities] (Brancourt 2020). Invoking a democracy of care on her blog in March 2020, lesbian, AIDS activist, and former member of ACT-UP Paris, Gwen Fauchois states "[l]es véritables experts de la réduction des risques et de la solidarité, c'est nous [communité sida] . . . nous devons d'abord apprendre à nous réunir, au moins provisoirement sans rassemblement physique" ["we [the AIDS community] are the true experts in risk reduction and solidarity practices . . . we must first learn to meet without a physical gathering, at least temporarily"] (Fauchois 2020a). Fauchois's comments are linked to Paul Preciado's (2020a) biotech understanding of epidemics as "de grands laboratoires d'innovation sociale, l'occasion d'une reconfiguration à grande échelle des techniques des corps et des technologies de pouvoir" ["large social innovation laboratories, the opportunity for a large-scale reconfiguration of techniques of the body and technologies of power"]. Indeed, framing pandemic protocols as opportunities for imagining novel biotech sexual solidarities and queer techno-kinship models allows us to reconsider the digitized circuit between the sex, sexual practices, sexual actors, and sexual citizenships produced during the pandemic as perhaps already a part of an inter-and transnational biotech economy of queer care in neoliberal times.

In London, for example, faced with the inability of sexual assemblage during their habitually held Sunday night SBN ("stark bollock naked") party, club organizers in Vauxhall went virtual connecting more than 3,000 participants within an erotic, biotech circuit of sexual subjectivities and praxes, a tenfold increase from pre-pandemic participation (Reid-Smith 2020). In France, the artistic and political project, *Erosticratie,* proposed a network of queer techno-kinship models and biotech sexual solidarities through its YouTube page and Skype allowing homebound adherents to communally listen to scheduled readings of "littérotique" ["erotic literature"], "erostocrate" ["individual user"] presentations of personal fetishes and novel sexual experiences, erotic virtual versions of "ASexMR" (autonomous sensory (sexual) meridian response), and to participate in virtual erotic group writing sessions (*Eristoconfinement* 2020). Finally, in an interview in *Remaides* in November 2020, Director of the association Acceptess-T and trans, sex-worker, and AIDS activist Giovanna Rincon traced the biotech circuits of queer care and solidarity for trans migrants, undocumented trans individuals, and sex workers who experience social mobility constraints, economic precarity, as well as larger, ongoing biopolitical discrimination exacerbated by SARS-CoV-2. Focusing on a democracy of care interwoven into inter-community networks of associative solidarity like the Facebook page "platforme de solidarités trans pédé gouine" ["trans fag dyke solidarity platform"],[16] Rincon states: "nous avons réalisé que [les mésures de réduction de risque proposées par le gouvernement] n'étaient pas adaptées aux personnes que l'on accompagnait . . . Nous avons mis en place toute une stratégie inter communautaire fondée sur la participation des personnes concernées et non sur le contrôle et la répression" ["we realized that the [risk-reduction measures put in place by the government] were not adapted to our center users . . . We put in place a whole inter-community strategy based on participation from those most impacted and not based on control or repression"] (Lebreton 2020, 22). Even with the expansive and relational mediatized circuit between HIV and SARS-CoV-2, these types of community-based networks of knowledge and interpersonal care mobilized during the AIDS crisis by queer activists remained largely liminal to state-sponsored approaches, protocols, and responses to the 2020 pandemic.

(UN)WILLED ADJACENCY: HIV AND SARS-COV-2

On 16 April 2020, Luc Montagnier, French virologist and joint recipient with Françoise Barré-Sinoussi and Harald zur Hausen of the Nobel Prize in Physiology or Medicine for the discovery of the human immunodeficiency virus (HIV), spoke with Jean-François Lemoine for a short interview on *Pourquoi Docteur: comprendre pour agir* [*Why Doctor: Information for Action*] revealing a newly emergent theory that etiologically linked HIV and SARS-CoV-2. Following genome sequencing that observed similarities between four pieces of genetic code in SARS-CoV-2 and genetic sequences found in certain HIV strains, Montagnier contended that the Wuhan laboratory, known according to his interview for its work on coronaviruses, was in the process of developing a future HIV vaccine when the newly constructed SARS-CoV-2, meant to serve as a vector for HIV antigens, would have escaped the lab through human intervention (Bietry 2020; *Pour le Pr Montagnier* 2020; Martin 2020). The biomedical underpinnings of Montagnier's postulate are perhaps at first glance innocuous: the spread of SARS-CoV-2 as an accidental world-altering event based in an ethics of global vaccinology. Such a claim, however, cannot be dislocated from coextensive national imaginings of SARS-CoV-2 in more nefarious terms, most notably as an intentionally manufactured bioweapon (Audureau 2020), linking it to historical, necropolitical conceptualizations of the emergence of HIV (Nattrass 2013, 114–120) and merging it with the hawkish epistemological framework of Macron's national address just a month prior. Indeed, allusions to SARS-CoV-2 as bioweaponry made by the *Pourquoi Docteur* interlocutor were never outright refuted by Montagnier during the interview, fueling at the very least accusations of bungled Chinese governmental biomedical policies and protocols already circulating in the international media following comments made by former Secretary of State Mike Pompeo, French President Emmanuel Macron, and former US President Donald Trump (Bietry 2020; "Coronavirus: Macron questions" 2020; Mallet and Roula 2020). Therefore, I title this section (un)willed adjacency to highlight the mutually constitutive epistemological and biopolitical circuit produced when HIV and SARS-CoV-2 are made proximate, a circuit that is formed by but also informs larger epistemological and biopolitical networks concerning conceptualizations of individual, community, nation, and citizenship.

To be sure, if many of these SARS-CoV-2 origin stories have by now been astutely challenged (Peron and Nieto 2020; Fact Check 2021),[17] it does not diminish the operational epistemological and biopolitical purchase that this (un)willed adjacency has created in media productions between bodies, desire, disease, and exception as can be seen in the citations that open the second section of this chapter. In their individual pandemic commentary, Seymet, Mazaurette, and Kraus all appeal to a discursive and temporal logics that brings HIV and SARS-CoV-2 into close proximity. They do so by questioning the current conditions of possibility for our own corporeal proximities through often specious analogies between past and present viro-existential circumstances, foregrounding relational epistemologies of loss, trauma, and sex that underscore the exceptional global precarity in which we exist as "living creatures . . . somatically interconnected by our body fluids" (Ljungcrantz and Gustavson 2020, 155). However, differing from the AIDS crisis when the possibility of seroconversion was associated almost exclusively with specific, outlying, epistemologically and socio-politically defined "risky" activities, bodies, and identities,[18] SARS-CoV-2 is understood as harboring the virological potential to affect all bodies, although to wildly varying degrees (Fassin 2020). In the cultural imaginary then, SARS-CoV-2 endues any-body with the potential to short-circuit entire global and local economic, sociopolitical, and sexual networks and systems, a devastatingly destructive, but also productive, biotechnology that might be understood through Sullivan and Murray's (2009) term "somatechnic" (21). Indeed, in an article in *Remaides*, Jean-François Laforgerie (2020) positions the month-long lockdown protocols in France as potential destructive/productive biotechnologies that might be mobilized to lower HIV infections through voluntary risk-reduction protocols and associative support:

> Ici, le "mois sans sexe" est un outil pour empêcher, dans une population donnée, la propagation du [VIH], en s'assurant que, pendant une période donnée, les personnes infectées et qui l'ignorent, seront diagnostiquées, se verront proposer un traitement ARV . . . et n'auront pas de rapports sexuels. Cette stratégie ne fonctionne que sur la base du volontariat et de la contrainte sociale acceptée. (24)
>
> [Here, the "month without sex" is a tool to prevent, in a given population, the propagation of [HIV], ensuring that, during a given period, the infected persons and those who do not know it, will be diagnosed, will be offered an ARV treatment . . . and will not have sex. This strategy only works if volitional and through acceptance of certain social constraints.]

The association AIDES digitized this biotech understanding of the productive/destructive possibilities of coming-out-of-lockdown through its June 2020 ludic, libidinous *lapin* [rabbit] campaign: a cheeky array of voyeuristic vignettes featuring sexually frustrated rabbits and catchy, shareable hashtags, #retrouvonsnousprotegeonsnous [#letsmeetupagainandprotecteachother] and #testbeforesex, all linked to informational associative networks providing an array of risk-reduction tools and protocols to accompany our long-awaited, post-lockdown sexual reunions (RetrouvonsNousProtegeonsNous 2020).

Given the exceptional biopolitical stakes of the pandemic, it is perhaps not so surprising to encounter the tropes of protection, safety, and war as impetus for action as in Macron's national call to citizens, Montagnier's interview, and Laforgerie's and the AIDES association's (post)lockdown risk-reduction protocols. In her classic work on AIDS, illness, and metaphors, Susan Sontag (2013) showed the historical efficacy of the operationalization of war lexicons for "mass ideological mobilization" campaigns against disease, often framed as emergencies "in which no sacrifice is excessive" (98–99), a discursive framework recently invoked by Emmanuel Macron in an interview on pandemic economics in *Financial Times* (2020). Although as Daniel Defert, co-founder of AIDES, points out, these calls for specific types of mobilization against disease are currently deployed mostly from the top down (state-centered response to SARS-CoV-2) rather than the bottom up (affected individual-centered response to HIV) (Favereau 2020). According to Paul Preciado (2020c), at the nexus of current (trans)national mobilization campaigns against the spread of SARS-CoV-2 is an immunological biopolitics operationalized at the national and individual levels. At the national level, this immunological biopolitics clarions the protection and fortification of socially constructed and defined national borders as the largely performative condition for guaranteeing national and individual biomedical integrity and safety. At the individual level, state immunological protocols are projected onto the bodies of individual citizens creating a synecdochic relation between breaches of individual epiderma-corporeal orifices and similar violations of communal/urban/national borders. The result is an overly simplistic, binary relation between inside/outside that makes almost all corporeal proximity and border transgressions biopolitically suspect. For Willy Rozenbaum, French physician and co-discoverer of HIV, current anxieties toward corporeal and therefore national and individual biomedical integrity and safety risk nourishing the bio-exclusionary frontier politics of the AIDS years, "sidatoriums," through today's pandemic lexicons, "coronatoriums" (Favereau 2020). Of course, as Preciado (2020d) reminds us, "Au temps du sida, il n'a donc pas été question de fermer les frontières. Il a été question de fermer l'anus" ["In the AIDS years there was no question of closing the borders, only talk of closing the anus"].[19]

Interrogating the biopolitical circuit between the individual and illness that forms and informs understandings of community and nation is important in these debates as etymological formulations of *immunity* and therefore immunitary biopolitics operate through a privative function: immunity is formed from the negation (*im*) of community *cum munus* (with duty). Preciado (2020c) explains: "The liberal and patriarchal-colonial European democracies of the nineteenth century constructed the ideal of the modern individual not only as a free economic agent (male, white, heterosexual) but also as an immunized body, radically separated, that owed nothing to the community." The bulk of Preciado's article traces past and present biopolitical technologies that, through appeals to state of exception protocols due to illness and disease, have worked in both Foucauldian and post-Foucauldian ways to fabricate, define, discipline, control, and operationalize different corporeal configurations and modes of being. Specifically, Preciado positions AIDS histories within the dynamic biotech circuits of knowledge/power networks and biotechnological management techniques that have informed past and current debates on the value and expendability of certain lives over others. Additionally, he invites us to consider (micro)political strategies informed by historical and epistemopolitical modes of understanding that might operationalize community and community knowledge against the necropolitical functioning of immunitary models of biopolitical life management. It is in this sense that the polysemic nature of the title of his article, "Learning from the virus," reveals all its exceptional semantic and prescient force because, of course, we can learn a great deal from the past and current experiences of individual and community activists when it comes to confronting epidemic disease at individual, communal, national, and global levels. Gwen Fauchois (2020a) made this point on her blog in March 2020, "s'il y a une communauté qui devrait partager son experience [à l'ère du Covid], c'est bien la communauté sida" ["if there's a community that should share its experience [during Covid times], it's the AIDS community"]. Indeed, opportunities for French officials to listen to this community have been prolific.

In their April 2020 letter to immunologist Jean-François Delfraissy and virologist Françoise Barré-Sinoussi responding to SARS-CoV-2 pandemic protocols in France that widely insulated economic interests to the detriment of the most precarized national populations, former ACT-UP Paris militants, members of Vers Paris sans sida [Toward AIDS-Free Paris], co-founders of the watchdog group l'Observatoire pour la transparence sur les politiques du medicament [Agency for Transparency on Drug Policies], and Giovanna Rincon, director of Acceptess-T, excavated in AIDS associative memory networks to underscore what we might learn from the revolutionary reversals in asymmetric biopolitical and biomedical knowledge/power dynamics from the beginning of the AIDS years: affected marginalized groups "ont revendiqué le savoir dont ils et elles étaient les dépositaires, ont imposé leur participation à la décision publique . . . se sont regroupés en associations et . . . [ont] construit la politique de lutte contre le sida" ["claimed the knowledge of which they were the custodians, imposed their participation in public decision-making . . . [,] came together in associations[,] and . . . built the policy to fight against AIDS"] ("Lettre Ouverte" 2020). A similar letter was signed by 26 queer associations and collectives in April calling on Marlène Schiappa, then secretary of state for gender equality, to adopt strategic risk-reduction measures mobilized by queer associations at the height of the AIDS years in order to better respond to the COVID-specific inequalities facing LGBTI+ individuals. The letter also suggested more generalized national policy possibilities based on community-based best practices from the fight against HIV ("Urgences LGBTI" 2020). An opinion piece in *Libération* in May 2020 made concurrent appeals ("Sortir du Covid-19 avec les citoyen.ne.s" 2020). Although as Aurélien Beaucamp, then president of the association AIDES, points out, even after recommendations made by Jean-François Delfraissy and Françoise Barré-Sinoussi to their own governmental health committees (Beaucamp 2020a, 5) these forms of democratic health services (*démocratie sanitaire*), including the creation of decision-making citizen committees (*comités citoyens*) in addition to scientific committees (Beaucamp 2020b), have been largely ignored by French health authorities in favor of more generalized, austere and neoliberal protocols and procedures informed by universalist benchmarks (white, male, heterosexual, middle-class) (Fauchois 2020b). Indeed, was it not a type of universalizing discursive amnesia that allowed French President Emmanuel Macron to announce in March 2020: "Le Covid-19 qui affecte tous les continents et frappe tous les pays européens est la plus grave crise sanitaire qu'ait connue la France depuis un siècle" ["Covid-19, which affects all continents and strikes all European countries, is the most serious health crisis in France for a century"] (Girard 2020)? The casual indifference of French government health officials to the expansive networks of sexual exception strategies offered through queer associative work is more than just necropolitical. Viewed through the mediatic juxtaposition of HIV and SARS-CoV-2 explored throughout this chapter, it might also be read as part of a larger economy of epistemological exploitation, appropriation, manipulation, and distortion of AIDS histories, discourses, and metaphors (Pézeril 2020).

CONCLUSION

There is something terribly ironic in the notion that exceptional (read: distinct and superior) sexual citizenship in COVID times was at least in part formed and informed by some of the very sexual practices and subjectivities that have exceptionally defined queer existence, and which have been historically relegated to undesirable if not anti-citizenship (Edelman 2004) or second-class citizenship (*citoyen de seconde zone*) (Le Bitoux, Proth, and Chevaux 2003) sexual positionings. As an always already existent sexual exception adaptable to the needs of pandemic times, queer conceptualizations of sexual citizenship created the conditions of possibility for generalized sexual actors to mitigate risk against illness, distance themselves from exposure to SARS-CoV-2, while simultaneously including them, through exception, in larger universalist citizenship circuits mobilized to protect the French nation.

In his reflection on the pandemic, Didier Lestrade (2021), author, journalist, and co-founder in 1989 of the Parisian branch of ACT-UP, reminds us that a type of sexual exception materialized at the height of the AIDS epidemic through changes in individual and community understandings of the circuit between sex, sexual citizenship, sexual practices, and risk reduction protocols as "[les] pratiques sexuelles étaient marquées par la peur des fluides corporels" ["sexual practices were marked by the fear of bodily fluids"]. Similar epistemological and biotech reconfigurations and reconceptualizations of this circuit are currently underway following the approval of pre-and post-exposure treatment options like PrEP in a variety of Western countries (Motta and Peetz 2019; Gomolka 2021). Perhaps, then, the current state of sexual exception is nothing new at all but rather a novel manifestation of an already existent epistemological and biotech circuit connecting and (re) defining sex, sexual citizenship, illness, individual, and nation dating back at the very least to the beginning of the HIV/AIDS crisis in France. Tracing a detailed genealogy of the dynamic, most certainly overlapping and mutually constitutive, manifestations of this circuit, would allow us to better understand the epistemologies and biotechnologies that are forming and informing current and future circuits between disease, sex, individual, and nation.

BIBLIOGRAPHY

Agamben, Giorgio. 2005. *The State of Exception*. Translated by Kevin Attell. Chicago: University of Chicago Press.

"Amour et sexe par temps de pandémie." 2021, *Arte: Tracks*, 11 February. https://www.arte.tv/fr/videos/100280-003-A/tracks/.

Anzaldúa, Gloria. 1987. *Borderlands/La Frontera: The New Mestiza*. San Francisco: Aunt Lute Books.

Audureau, William. 2020. "Le coronavirus, « arme biologique »? Le vrai du faux d'une vidéo virale." *Le Monde*, 6 March. https://www.lemonde.fr/les-decodeurs/article/2020/03/06/le-coronavirus-arme-biologique-le-vrai-du-faux-d-une-video-virale_6032098_4355770.html.

Audureau, William, Jonathan Parienté, Mathilde Damgé, and Assma Maad. 2021. "Passe sanitaire: où sera-t-il exigé à partir de lundi? A qui s'applique-t-il? Les résponses à vos questions." *Le Monde*, 13 July. https://www.lemonde.fr/les-decodeurs/article/2021/07/13/passe-sanitaire-ou-sera-t-il-exige-quels-tests-seront-acceptes-les-questions-que-pose-son-extension_6088173_4355770.html.

Beaucamp, Aurélien. 2020a. "Questions de confiance!" *REMAIDES: VIH, Covid-19 la face masquée de discrimination*, no 113 (novembre): 4–5. https://www.aides.org/remaides/remaides-113-disponible.

———. 2020b. Interview by Pablo Vivien-Pillaud and Pierre Jacquemain. *La Midinale*. 30 November, http://www.regards.fr/la-midinale/article/aurelien-beaucamp-il-y-a-une-discrimination-institutionnalisee-des-personnes.

Bell, David and Jon Binnie. 2000. *The Sexual Citizen: Queer Politics and Beyond.* Malden: Blackwell Publishers.

Bierty, Guillaume. 2020. "Coronavirus et VIH: pourquoi la théorie du Pr Montagnier est très contestable" *Têtu*, 19 avril. https://tetu.com/2020/04/19/coronavirus-et-vih-pourquoi-la-theorie-du-pr-montagnier-est-tres-contestable/.

Brancourt, Mathieu. 2020. "Covid-19 et VIH: le vent se (re)lève?" *REMAIDES: VIH et Covid-19 Que sait-on?*, no. 111 (avril): 38–41. https://www.aides.org/remaides/remaides-111-disponible.

Butler, Judith. 2011."Precarious Life: The Obligations of Proximity." Lecture, Nobel Prize Museum, Svenska Akademiens Börssal, May 24, https://www.youtube.com/watch?v=KJT69AQtDtg.

Cole, Anaïs. 2020. "La Covid-19 est devenue un frein à la liberté sexuelle des célibataires." *Pourquoi Docteur: comprendre pour agir*, 20 juillet. https://www.pourquoidocteur.fr/Articles/Question-d-actu/33262-La-Covid-19-devenue-frein-liberte-sexuelle-celibataires.

"Coronavirus: la sexualité confinée." *SudOuest*, 20 March. https://www.sudouest.fr/sante/coronavirus-la-sexualite-confinee-2020168.php.

"Coronavirus: Macron Questions China's Handling of Outbreak." 2020. *BBC*, 17 April, https://www.bbc.com/news/world-europe-52319462.

Crimp, Douglas. 1989. "Mourning and Militancy." *October* 51 (winter): 3–18.

Cvetkovich, Anne. 2003. *An Archive of Feeling: Trauma, Sexuality, and Lesbian Public Cultures*. Durham: Duke UP.

Dunbar, Willy. 2020. "Le Covid-19 suscite une nouvelle stigmatization des personnes LGBT+." *The Conversation*, 14 mai. https://theconversation.com/le-covid-19-suscite-une-nouvelle-stigmatisation-des-personnes-lgbt-138159.

De Charette, Laurence. 2021. "Covid-19 et natalité, les enfants oubliés." *Le Figaro*, 11 mars. https://www.lefigaro.fr/actualite-france/covid-19-et-natalite-les-enfants-oublies-20210311.

Diallo, Rokhaya. 2020. "France on Lockdown: Vacation for Some, a Nightmare for Many." *Aljazeera*, 19 April. https://www.aljazeera.com/opinions/2020/4/10/france-on-lockdown-vacation-for-some-a-nightmare-for-many.

Diallo, Rokhaya and Jérémy Robine. 2020. "En Seine-Saint-Denis, le virus de la ségrégation raciale." 7 May, https://www.liberation.fr/debats/2020/05/07/en-seine-saint-denis-le-virus-de-la-segregation-raciale_1787705/.

Duranton, Julia. 2020. "Sexe et Covid: la pratique du Glory Hole conseillée par les autorités sanitaires." *Cosmopolitan*, 29 juillet. https://www.cosmopolitan.fr/sexe-pendant-l-epidemie-de-coronavirus-l-usage-du-glory-hole-conseille,2036855.asp.

Durin-Valois, Marc. 2020. "Sex and the Covid: l'amour entre puritanisme et «glory hole»." *Mediapart*. 4 novembre. https://blogs.mediapart.fr/marc-durin-valois/blog/041120/sex-and-covid-l-amour-entre-puritanisme-et-glory-hole.

Edelman, Lee. 2004. *No Future: Queer Theory and the Death Drive*. Durham: Duke University Press.

Erostocratie. n.d. "Eristoconfinement." Accessed May 18, 2020. https://www.erosticratie.fr/erosticonfinement.

"Fact Check: SARS-CoV-2 Was Not Created Using Genes from HIV, Fauci Does Not Hold Patents for an 'HIV Component' to SARS-CoV-2." 2021. *Reuters*, 7 January. https://www.reuters.com/article/uk-factcheck-hiv-covid-explained/fact-check-SARS-CoV-2 -was-not-created-using-genes-from-hiv-fauci-does-not-hold-patents-for-an-hiv-component-to-SARS-CoV-2 -idUSKBN29C26E.

Fassin, Didier. 2020. "L'illusion dangereuse de l'égalité devant l'épidémie." *College de France*, 16 April. https://www.college-de-france.fr/site/didier-fassin/L-illusion-dangereuse-de-legalite-devant-lepidemie.htm.

Fauchois, Gwen. 2020a. "Coronavirus: La réduction des risques et la solidarité, c'est nous." *Gwen Fauchois* (blog). *Blogspot.com.* 12 mars. http://gwenfauchois.blogspot.com/2020/03/.

———. 2020b. "Coronavirus: la réduction des risques, c'est encore et toujours nous." *Mediapart*, 25 avril. https://blogs.mediapart.fr/gwen-fauchois/blog/250420/coronavirus-la-reduction-des-risques-cest-encore-et-toujours-nous.

Favereau, Eric. 2020. "Chronique 'Aux petits soins' Sida et Covid-19: 'Aujourd'hui, c'est un peu la même inconnue.'" *Libération*, 7 avril. https://www.liberation.fr/france/2020/04/07/sida-et-covid-19-aujourd-hui-c-est-un-peu-la-meme-inconnue_1784367/.

Giami, A. 2021. "COVID-19 et sexualités: l'émergence d'un nouveau paradigme des sexualités COVID-19 and sexualities: The emergence of a new paradigm of sexualities." *Sexologies*, vol. 30, issue 1 (mars). https://www.sciencedirect.com/science/article/pii/S1158136021000025?via%3Dihub.

Giard, Agnès. 2020. "Faire l'amour par un trou?" *Libération*, 7 septembre. https://www.liberation.fr/debats/2020/09/07/faire-l-amour-par-un-trou_1811131/.

Girard, Gabriel. 2020. "Covid-19: quelques leçons de la lute contre le VIH/sida." *Medium*, 27 May. https://medium.com/@GbrlGirard/covid-19-quelques-leçons-de-la-lutte-contre-le-vih-sida-1a25a25ba76b.

Gomolka, CJ. 2019. "(Don't) Call Me Queer: Transpédégouine, the Global Gay, and the Logics of Western 'Liberty.'" *Contemporary French Civilization*, vol 44, number 4: 417–433.

———. 2021. "The Queer Aesthetics of la PrEP: Iconography, the Pharmac opornographic Regime, and (Safe) Sex in the French Neoliberal Marketplace." *Contemporary French Civilization*, vol 46, number 2.

Grenoble, Ryan. 2021. "Fauci Addresses Reports of Ill Wuhan Researchers, COVID Lab Theory." *Huffpost*, 24 May. https://www.huffpost.com/entry/fauci-covid-lab-animal_n_60ac0db7e4b0d56a83ed172a.

"Health Equity Considerations and Racial and Ethnic Minority Groups." 2021. *CDC*, 19 April. https://www.cdc.gov/coronavirus/2019-ncov/community/health-equity/race-ethnicity.html.

Kraus, François. 2020. "La vie sexuelle des français déconfinés grande frousse ou grand relâchement?: Enquête sur l'activité sexuelle des Français depuis la fin du confinement." *IFOP*, juillet. https://www.ifop.com/publication/la-vie-sexuelle-des-francais-deconfines-grande-frousse-ou-grand-relachement/.

"L'activité sexuelle des Français a quasiment retrouvé son niveau d'avant la crise sanitaire, malgré le reconfinement." 2020. *Franceinfo*. 9 décembre. https://www.francetvinfo.fr/sante/maladie/coronavirus/confinement/l-activite-sexuelle-des-francais-a-quasiment-retrouve-son-niveau-d-avant-la-crise-sanitaire-malgre-le-reconfinement_4212923.html.

Laforgerie, Jean-François. 2020. "Le confinement, un outil contre le VIH?" *Remaides*, no. 111 (avril): 23–27. https://www.aides.org/remaides/remaides-111-disponible.

Laubier, Charles de. 2020. "La fracture numérique au révélateur du Covid-19." *Le Monde*, 30 August, https://www.lemonde.fr/economie/article/2020/08/30/la-fracture-numerique-au-revelateur-du-covid-19_6050380_3234.html.

Le Bitoux, Jean, Bruno Proth and Hervé Chevaux. 2003. *Citoyen de seconde zone: trente ans de lutte pour la reconnaissance de l'homosexualité en France (1971–2002)*. Paris: Hachette.

Lebreton, Fred. 2020. "Giovanna Rincon: 'Cette crise a été un grand tsunami pour la communauté trans.'" *Remaides*, no. 113 (novembre): 21–23. https://www.aides.org/remaides/remaides-113-disponible.

Leclair, Angès. 2021. "Natalité perturbée par le Covid-19: la baisse des naissances s'atténue en février." *Le Figaro*, 26 mars. https://www.lefigaro.fr/actualite-france/natalite-perturbee-par-le-covid-19-la-baisse-des-naissances-s-attenue-en-fevrier-20210326.

Lestrade, Didier. 2021. "La 'vie d'avant.'" *Didier Lestrade* (blog), 25 janvier. http://didierlestrade.blogspot.com/2021/01/la-vie-davant.html.

"Lettre ouverte à Françoise Barré-Sinoussi et Jean-François Delfraissy." 2020. *Mediapart*, 7 avril. https://blogs.mediapart.fr/edition/les-invites-de-mediapart/article/070420/lettre-ouverte-francoise-barre-sinoussi-et-jean-francois-delfraissy.

Ljungcrantz, Desireé and Malena Gustavson, 2020. "HIV and the Somatechnics of Viral Networks, Temporalities and Politics": *Somatechnics*, vol. 10, no. 2 (august): pp. 155–171.

Macron, Emmanuel. 2020. "Discours du 16, mars 2020." *Youtube*, 16 mars. https://www.youtube.com/watch?v=mhklV9uOvTQ.

Mallet, Victor and Roula Khalaf. 2020. "FT Interview: Emmanuel Macron Says It Is Time to Think the Unthinkable." *Financial Times*, 16 April. https://www.ft.com/content/3ea8d790-7fd1-11ea-8fdb-7ec06edeef84.

Manière, Pierre. 2018. "Accès à Internet: de fortes disparités au-delà du périphérique parisien." *La Tribune*, 27 juin. https://www.latribune.fr/technos-medias/internet/acces-a-internet-de-fortes-disparites-au-dela-du-peripherique-783164.html.

Martin, Nicolas. 2020. "Un lien entre Covid-19 et VIH?" *France Culture*, 17 avril. https://www.franceculture.fr/emissions/radiographies-du-coronavirus/un-lien-entre-covid-19-et-vih.

Mazaurette, Maïa. 2020. "Coronavirus: cet été, sexualité rimera avec austerité." *Le Monde*, 24 mai. https://www.lemonde.fr/m-perso/article/2020/05/24/covid-19-cet-ete-sexualite-rimera-avec-austerite_6040564_4497916.html.

Motta, Carlos, and John Aurthur Peetz. 2019. "Because PrEP Is Not about AIDS: An Exchange to Expand on the PrEP Manifesto between Carlos Motta and John Arthur Peetz," *Oncurating*, Issue 42 (September): 132–140, https://www.on-curating.org/

files/oc/dateiverwaltung/issue42/PDF_to_Download/OnCurating_Issue_42_Web.pdf.

Natrass, Nicoli. 2013. "Understanding the Origins and Prevalence of AIDS Conspiracy Beliefs in the United States and South Africa." *Sociology of Health and Illness*, vol 35, no 1: 113–129. https://onlinelibrary-wiley-com.duproxy.palni.edu/doi/pdfdirect/10.1111/j.1467-9566.2012.01480.x.

"Oui, le vaccin peut avoir des effets désirables: vaccinons-nous!" 2021. *Agence régionale de santé Provence-Alpes Côte d'Azur*. 24 June. https://www.paca.ars.sante.fr/oui-le-vaccin-peut-avoir-des-effets-desirables-vaccinons-nous.

Papon, Sylvain and Catherine Beaumel. 2021. "Bilan démographique 2020: Avec la pandémie de Covid-19, nette baisse de l'espérance de vie et chute du nombre de mariages." *Institut national de la statistique et des études économiques*, 19 janvier. https://www.insee.fr/fr/statistiques/5012724.

Peron, Iris and Sébastien Neito. 2020. "Coronavirus et VIH: pourquoi la théorie du Pr Luc Montagnier est invraisemblable." *Le Parisien,* 17 avril. https://www.leparisien.fr/societe/coronavirus-et-vih-pourquoi-la-theorie-du-pr-luc-montagnier-est-invraisemblable-17-04-2020-8301387.php.

Pézeril, Charlotte. 2020. "Du Sida au Covid-19: Les leçons de la lutte contre le VIH." *La Vie des Idées*, 2 octobre. https://laviedesidees.fr/Du-Sida-au-Covid-19.html.

"Pour le Pr Montagnier, SARS-CoV-2 serait un virus manipulé par les Chinois avec de l'ADN de VIH!" 2020. *Pourquoi docteur*, 16 avril. https://www.pourquoidocteur.fr/Articles/Question-d-actu/32184-EXCLUSIF-Pour-Pr-Montagnier-SARS-CoV-2-serait-virus-manipule-Chinois-l-ADN-de-VIH-podcast.

Preciado, Paul. 2013. *Testo Junkie: Sex, Drugs, and Biopolitics in the Pharmacopornographic Era*. Translated by Bruce Benderson. New York: The Feminist Press.

———. 2020a. "Biosurveillance: sortir de la prison molle de nos intérieurs." *Mediapart*, 12 avril. https://www.mediapart.fr/journal/international/120420/biosurveillance-sortir-de-la-prison-molle-de-nos-interieurs?onglet=full.

———. 2020b. "Corona fashion." *Libération*, 8 mai. https://www.liberation.fr/debats/2020/05/08/corona-fashion_1787839/.

———. 2020c. "Learning from the Virus." *Artforum,* mai/juin. https://www.artforum.com/print/202005/paul-b-preciado-82823.

———. 2020d. "Le Brexit et mon lumbago," *Libération,* 1 mars.

Preston, Julia. 2009. "Obama Lifts a Ban on Entry into U.S. by H.I.V.-Positive People." *The New York Times*, 30 October. https://www.nytimes.com/2009/10/31/us/politics/31travel.html.

Provencher, Denis M. 2007. *Queer French: Globalization, Language, and Sexual Citizenship in France*. New York: Routledge.

Puar, Jasbir. 2007. *Terrorist Assemblages: Homonationalism in Queer Times*. Durham: Duke UP.

Rauglaudre, Timothée de. 2020. "Pour ces leaders religieux, le coronavirus est une punition divine contre l'homosexualité." *Têtu*, 10 mars. https://tetu.com/2020/03/10/pour-ces-leaders-religieux-le-coronavirus-est-une-punition-divine-contre-lhomosexualite/.

Reid-Smith, Tris. 2020. "A Gay Sex Club Has Taken Its Naked Party Online and Proved More Popular Than Ever." *GSN*, 30 March. https://www.gaystarnews.com/article/a-gay-sex-club-has-taken-its-naked-party-online-and-proved-more-popular-than-ever/.

"RetrouvonsNousProtegeonsNous: AIDES et son agence TBWA invitent à protéger nos retrouvailles du VIH et des IST." 2020. *AIDES*, 5 juin. https://www.aides.org/sites/default/files/Aides/bloc_telechargement/CP%20reveal%20%23RetrouvonsNousProtegeonsNous.pdf.

"Safer Sex and COVID-19." 2020. *NYC Health Department*, 8 June. https://www1.nyc.gov/assets/doh/downloads/pdf/imm/covid-sex-guidance.pdf.

Samourcachian, Elisa. 2020. "Pour se protéger du covid, les autorités canadiennes conseillent le 'glory hole.'" *Huffpost*, 27 July. https://www.huffingtonpost.fr/entry/les-autorites-canadiennes-recommandent-le-glory-hole-pour-eviter-toute-transmission-du-virus-pendant-un-rapport_fr_5f1ea259c5b638cfec47451d.

"Sexe et amours confinés." 2020. *RTS*, 11 juin. https://www.rts.ch/play/tv/temps-present/video/sexe-et-amours-confines--le-pire-match-de-ma-vie?urn=urn:rts:video:11393855.

"Sexe et pandémie: «Les activités sexuelles les moins risquées pendant que sévit la Covid-19 sont celles où vous êtes seul." 2020. *Courrier-Picard*, 3 septembre. https://www.courrier-picard.fr/id124576/article/2020-09-03/sexe-et-pandemie-au-canada-le-port-du-masque-suggere-pour-certains-couples.

Seymat, Thomas. 2020. "Sexe, drague et coronavirus: comment se protéger à l'heure de Covid-19." *Euronews*, 23 mars. https://fr.euronews.com/2020/03/23/relations-sexuelles-drague-comment-se-proteger-a-l-heure-du-coronavirus.

Sikouk, Bessma. 2020. "Moins de sexe mais plus d'expérimentations pendant le confinement." *Slate.fr*, 29 juillet. http://www.slate.fr/story/193116/sexualite-confinement-covid-19-relations-sexuelles-nouvelles-pratiques.

Sontag, Susan. 2013. *Illness as Metaphor and AIDS and Its Metaphors*. Picador. Kindle.

"Sortir du Covid-19 avec les citoyen·ne·s." 2020. *Libération*, 6 May. https://www.liberation.fr/debats/2020/05/06/sortir-du-covid-19-avec-les-citoyennes_1787538/.

Sullivan, Nikki, and Samantha Murray, Samantha, eds. 2009. *Somatechnics: Queering Technologisation of Bodies*, London: Taylor & Francis.

Tanguy, Youen. 2020. "Les jeunes LGBT+, victimes collatérales de la crise du Covid-19." *Komitid*, 20 avril. https://www.komitid.fr/2020/04/20/les-jeunes-lgbt-victimes-collaterales-de-la-crise-du-covid-19/.

"Urgences LGBTQI Durant le confinement: lettre à Marlène Schiappa." 2020. *AIDES*, 28 avril. https://www.aides.org/communique/urgences-lgbtqi-durant-le-confinement-lettre-marlene-schiappa.

Vallaud-Belkacem, Najat and Sandra Laugier. 2020. *La société des vulnérables: leçons féministes d'une crise*. Paris: Éditions Gallimard. Kindle.

Valo, Martine. 2021. "La pandémie de Covid-19 a créé un « baby flop » mondial." *Le Monde*, 4 avril. https://www.lemonde.fr/international/article/2021/04/04/la-pandemie-de-covid-19-a-cree-un-bebe-flop-mondial_6075514_3210.html.

Viala, Océane. 2021. "Entre vibros et visios, voici à quoi ressemblent vos sexualités confinées." *Mademoizelle*, 27 janvier. https://www.madmoizelle.com/sexe-a-distance-confinement-1048957.

NOTES

1. For information on France see Vallaud-Belkacem and Laugier 2020 and Diallo and Robine 2020; for general information see "Health Equity" 2021.

2. Unless otherwise indicated, all translations are my own.

3. These headlines come from *Huffpost*, *France Culture*, and *SudOuest*, respectively.

4. While beyond the scope of this contribution, we might consider the recent implementation of the "passe sanitaire" (health pass) in France and the Schengen zone as intimately linked to notions of biotechsex. Current French national protocols require the scanning of individual QR codes on cellphones, that link to an individual's vaccination or COVID-test status as attested through the national health system, in order to freely enter spaces of (sexual) sociality like bars, clubs, restaurants, (movie) theaters, and sports clubs (Audureau 2021). In this formulation, the cellphone becomes a type of biotech prosthesis that attests to the health of the body while also inserting the body into a digitized transactional circuit of national and capitalist health and monetary interest. In addition to its disciplinary implications, the health pass also seems to rewrite social scripts and citizenship models, QR codes becoming the new (a)social form of salutation and proof, or not, of national health and "good" citizenship compliancy models.

5. Agamben speaks specifically of the shifting status of individuals suspected of terrorists acts after 9/11 and of Jewish individuals during WWII.

6. Gloria Anzaldúa (1987) theorizes the notion of "rigidity" in her critical conceptualization of *la mestiza* going as far as suggesting that "[r]igidity means death" (79). In the context of this chapter, rigid formulations of sexuality and sexual citizenship that lead to little or no sex could indeed be necropolitical.

7. Preciado defines pharmacopornographic as referring to "the processes of a biomolecular (pharmaco) and semiotic-technical (pornographic) government of sexual subjectivity" (33–4). For Preciado this regime functions by activating cycles of "excitation-frustration" (275) integrating bodies into a larger pharmacoporn economy that runs on and mobilizes the collective desires and "ejaculatory capital" (50) of all sexual citizens.

8. A city, the author states, still haunted by AIDS epidemic.

9. See also Kraus 2020.

10. Here, I am modifying a formulation presented by Judith Butler (Butler 2011) from a talk given at the Nobel Prize Museum on precarious life.

11. "Confinement" was one of the terms used in France for "lockdown."

12. Most media contributions during this period insist on the state of sexual exception by creating a visual tension and contingency in their titles between "sex" and "pandemic": "Sexe et pandémie" (sex and pandemic), "Safer-sex and COVID-19," "COVID-19 and Sex."

13. Macron adds "en temps de paix" (in peacetimes) while simultaneously speaking of being "en guerre" (at war).

14. Via a German documentary, *Arte* "Tracks" dedicated a 30-minute episode to the ways that sex workers, escorts, and individual pornographic filmmakers were innovating during the pandemic (*Amour et sexe*); similarly, RTS dedicated an episode examining the reconceptualizing of love and sex during the pandemic entitled, "Sexe et amours confinés."

15. See also Laubier 2020.

16. For more information on the history and circulation of the term "transpédégouine" see Gomolka 2019.

17. In May 2021, understandings of the etiology of the virus as man-made in Wuhan resurfaced and deserve, according to Dr. Anthony Fauci, "thorough investigation" (Grenoble 2021).

18. Often mnemonically indexed as the 4 Hs: homosexuals, Haitians, hemophiliacs, and heroin users.

19. Preciado is speaking here from a European perspective. There was, in fact, a 22-year ban on travel to the United States for seropositive individuals lifted in 2009 by then President Obama (see Preston 2009).

Chapter Eight

Interview with Nicholas Giguère and Kevin Lambert

John Ashburn and Loïc Bourdeau

Nicholas Giguère (NG) and Kevin Lambert (KL) are two millennial queer writers from Quebec, Canada, who have each published a number of critically acclaimed queer, raw books. In this interview, we discuss their relationship with rawness, writing, queerness, contemporary (gay) sociality, and HIV/AIDS.

JA & LB: Your works make much room for violence, queer identity, and sexuality and desire. To what extent is the literary space a place to explore rawness and are there limits to this kind of writing?

NG: Our current moment, I think, is perhaps more than ever open to rawness: it allows for several authors to explore questions of sexuality and to speak (about oneself) without hiding behind obscure metaphors, coded references, or what I would call more generally, the thickness of language. Rawness then becomes a way to define oneself in a direct manner. As for limits, I don't believe there are any limits to raw writing—at least, I don't want to give it any. I'm ready to go as far as possible in the shamelessness, the unveiling, even if I don't necessarily value myself, even if what I write about myself is degrading, even if I endanger myself. In fact, writing is always a form of exposition to danger, and it is that risk that I want to find in the works that I read, in the books that I write.

KL: You would have to define this strange word "rawness." It's an ambiguous term, which in the current language is opposed to "cooked" (one thinks of the title of Levi-Strauss' work). According to an online dictionary it also means: "direct, brutal." These two definitions imply a sort of naturality and authenticity. Is raw the primordial state of that which is only presented to us in a cooked manner? What does that tell us about "cooked" books? The raw also recalls the old opposition, often deconstructed, between nature and culture: It's a meat metaphor (the etymology takes us back to "blood") that speaks of books as if they were steaks. In everyday language, "raw" tends to come loaded with moral judgment. The things that are said to be raw (or crude) are the ones that deviate from the "acceptable," whether it be a parent's crude jokes that children mustn't hear or films that are rated R because they contain sex scenes. Rawness points to situations where what shouldn't be said, done, or seen comes up in sanitized or regulated places. To be honest, I struggle to accept this notion for two reasons. On the one hand, it seems to me that rawness implies a kind of intrinsic naturalness—the raw as an earlier state, almost pre-cultural—and, on the other, because this notion is predominantly used as a moral judgment in a world where the "acceptable" would otherwise reign. Who defines or decides what's acceptable? I guess that in my books, the raw is everything that is traditionally perceived as "taboo" (sex, suicide, physical aggression, etc.). However, in my writing, I often try to put an end to these taboos; fiction can give new meaning to realities or experiences that are usually seen in a negative light. For example, *Querelle de Roberval* (2018) ends with a scene of cannibalism. Absolute taboo! But I wanted to write it in a very "casual" way on purpose, without casting judgment on it. You see the employees cooking their boss as if it were something they did daily, and no one finds it shocking. In the realm of fiction, cannibalism becomes comical; it's playing on the expression "eat the rich." As such, I'm not sure that this "raw" subject is very raw anymore.

JA & LB: Raw writing is direct, without detour. Queer(ness) is perhaps more of a deviation, the avoidance of a direct path (*straight*). It seems that your writing is at once raw and queer.

NG: I think it's possible to define queerness in many ways: it's a vast theory, an expansive approach. For me, queerness is anything but a deviation, a form of avoidance: it's more a frontal and incisive critique of the direct path that is *straightitude*, a reassessment of all the rigid standard categories. In my life, this criticism happens most notably in brutal and visceral writing. For me, queer and raw go hand in hand.

KL: Like Nicholas, I think "straight" culture is often a culture of avoidance, of the unsaid, the illicit, and the repressed. What is designated as queer *can* refer to the baroque (e.g., interlacing, decoration, fake). But, it can also imply a more "direct" relation to desires, sexuality, or a long-refused identity. I've actually been reading Proust and I'm quite fascinated by how these different aesthetics coexist. In the "straight" world that Proust creates, homosexuality is despised, taboo, secret, but at the same time, everyone knows his secret and everyone pretends not to see it. *Straight* characters allude to Charlus's homosexuality or rely on paraphrases to do so. Yet, in the end, they all turn out to be quite queer . . .

JA & LB: Your writing seems to attack neoliberalism, capitalism, consumerism, and heteropatriarchy directly. Is that so? Do you have a specific readership in mind?

NG: Any writer who claims to have no reader in mind when writing is either a hypocrite or totally clueless. In essence, literature, which can be defined in different ways, depending on one's standpoint, is an act of communication as Roman Jakobson understood it: literature needs readers to exist. I hope to talk to people who are looking for new discourses on male homosexuality—discourses (and even representations) they can identify with or relate to. I want these discourses and representations to be critical of heteronormativity, toxic masculinity, and androcentrism, all of which still poison our societies and imageries. How many problems are caused by people—namely men—who believe they can do however they please? I've had enough of the impunity of men obsessed with their privileges. It is the nature of literature to say it and *bring about something* else. And that "something else" must not be the result of a pre-established program. Literature is not programmatic.

KL: For me, it's not so much about readership as much as it is about personal considerations. It's about what I've lived, what I'm living, what worries me, interests me, and mobilizes me from day to day. That's why I talk about it in my work. These concepts you mention in your question are heavy: they are so talked about that they lose meaning. At any rate, in fiction, I don't work with concepts. Of course, I read and stay informed on all of these subjects, but in life, how often does one encounter "heteropatriarchy" in the street? We experience its symbols, its incarnations, the concrete consequences of its logic on people's lives. Literature interests me because it thinks, in a sense, beyond the concept. Where a scholar would need to define its terms at length, to inscribe them into a larger history, and would, in turn, rely on all-encompassing concepts that remove complexity, plurality, and multitude, fiction needs not ask itself how to name the superstructures that frame different phenomena of domination and exploitation. It speaks of all of that without having to generalize. I try to work on the human terrain, psychology, and experiences. I ask myself: How do the people, who don't think like me, think? How is one, at a human level, a capitalist, a sexist, a racist, a homophobe? How do these logics function concretely, and how do those who are submitted to them perceive them? How do they interact with one another? On which texts and social discourses are they based? Literature can accomplish a lot by complexifying, adding to, or blurring our political understanding, all while approaching "politics" in a more lively and embodied way.

JA & LB: HIV and AIDS are present in your works (through bodily fluids and the attendant historical trauma). What does this imagery bring to your writing? What does it say about gay sociality in the 21st century?

NG: I cannot write and lose sight of those—primarily men—who preceded me and who, in the worst of the crisis, in the 1980s and 1990s, literally waged an all-out war against HIV and AIDS. Many have died fighting, too. Tragically so. We must not forget them, pretend they never existed. I don't mean to come across as judgmental, but it seems that some authors do not acknowledge this debt: they present HIV/AIDS as if it were a "chronic illness" we can cure with tritherapy or prevent with the holy PrEP. There is an entire history behind HIV/AIDS, and this historicization is missing in some works. It is important to have HIV/AIDS discourses that are always anchored in lived experiences.

KL: Some discourse insists on making AIDS an "era" (as bygone), a sort of archaic remains. When one lives in the vicinity of "gayness" today, or if one has even the slightest idea of the international situation, it is evident that AIDS is anything but the "past." The worst of the epidemic—and what it revealed and set in motion in society is—barely behind us. As Nicholas says, many people should still be alive today, still creating performances and writing books, playing in the movies. I feel their absent words, their lost voices. We don't know, and we may never know all that we have lost. We have yet to truly fathom the symbolic and imaginary dimension of AIDS, which largely preceded it too. The ideas of disease, of contamination, of condemnation, of the manifestation of a fundamental flaw, of the concretization of sin, of a potentially fatal secret, have all been strongly linked to the epidemic. Today, though, these ideas still have an effect on queer imagination, on the relations between gays and straights, and homophobic discourse, for example.

The ongoing COVID-19 crisis, which has affected different populations, caused different symptoms, and led to a swifter governmental response, has given many the impression of a replayed epidemic. The cruel irony now is that those who were under attack during the AIDS epidemic in the 1980s and 1990s are now the most at risk of dying from COVID-19 (because of their age). But at any rate, COVID is already over, isn't it? Are we not in "the post-covid world" already? Like Nicholas, I think in writing, I try to preserve a form of memory of the presence of AIDS, its traumas and fantasies.

JA & LB: It seems that rawness allows for the (re)valorization of sexuality, particularly non-heterosexuality. Are you trying to reach a form of normalization?

NG: Not at all. I've always used writing to say, name, and reclaim my sexuality in all its dimensions, but never to normalize it. "Normalizing a specific sexuality," for me, is to categorize it, classify it and force it into tiny boxes—often there is only one box—to objectify it, reduce to it to a few stereotypical traits. To smother it. Literature must never seek to normalize anything at all. Because if it does, it becomes something that is no longer literature.

The idea of "normal" actually needs to be completely reevaluated. It's what queerness teaches us: to doubt constructed categories like "man," "woman," "masculine," "feminine," "gay," etc., and to distrust theoretical shortcuts.

KL: Raw is really like "trash," a moral and aesthetic judgment placed on the representation of non-heterosexuality. For most people, *Querelle de Roberval* was "trash" because the protagonist sodomizes young men on the first page (lots of people didn't read any further).

I share Virginie Despentes' reading of the social world in *King Kong théorie*, where she explains that we live in a hypocritical world that sells sex everywhere in advertisements and cinema, but at the same time cloaks it in taboo, banishing it to the realm of the irrepresentable, the unsayable. For this reason, sex automatically has a transgressive aura when it appears in art. Everyone watches pornography. Its consumption is based in large part on a libidinal logic. Still, conscientious parents are staunchly against teaching sexual education in school. In books like in university seminars, or among friends, we never speak of sexuality, at least not too explicitly. And if we do talk about it, it is to say, "how crude!" We are still in very puritan societies when it comes to attraction, pleasure, fantasy, sodomy, sex with no phallus or with objects, domination and submission play, etc. This taboo affects heterosexuality, even if it is more widespread and visible. Apparently, sex should not be talked about or shown and writers interested in it are nothing but perverts.

The question about normalization is important: there is quite a strong call for queer writers to propose "positive representations," lessons of hope that, quite often, correspond to the social order in place and heterosexist narratives—"we aren't in 1950 anymore," "we're making progress," "what you do in the bedroom isn't any of my concern," "gays, trans, lesbians, are just like everyone else," "we need more members of the LGBTQ community in office." I look forward to a time when literature is free of this constant frame of reading that always boils down to "representations" (positive or negative). This frame certainly has its pertinence for me when dealing with mainstream or children's cinema. That said, there is, however, a trap in wanting to avoid any form of "normalization" at all costs. For example, I wouldn't wish for LGBTQ authors to be afraid of negative feedback for writing characters or relationships that are too "normalized" or "replicating codes of heterosexuality" (Butler deconstructed the idea in *Gender Trouble*) as if that would ruin the "purity" of their queerness! Given today's lack of non-heterosexual and non-cisgender poetics and aesthetics, maybe what should be undone is our quickness to draw our judgments, our tendency to classify works as correct or incorrect, too much or not "normalized" enough, problematic or not, to actually start to really read them.

JA & LB: You choose geographic spaces that are also raw and/or violent. How do these spaces affect individuals? Could you also speak on the dichotomy between big cities and rural cities that seems to influence your imagination?

NG: In *Queues* (2017), I speak about gay bars in particular, which I've always found violent. I recognize that these are important spaces of sociality and that they served as safe spaces at a specific time, but I never felt comfortable there. The regulars who look at the newly arrived with starving eyes, the cliques it's difficult, even impossible, to join, the side eyes, the judgment: all of this disgusts me. In a bar, I feel like a piece of meat and nothing else. This toxicity is also perceptible on dating sites and applications. It's what I showed, I think, with *Petites annonces* (2020), a book I wrote based on ads from real profiles that revealed the existence of several forms of discrimination within the LGBTQ+ community: racism, fatphobia, ageism, classism, hatred of effeminacy, the fetishization of racialized and trans persons, etc.

I also depicted the countryside as a violent space, particularly in *Quelqu'un* (2018). I am from a rural region myself. I experienced discrimination in high school because of my physique, good grades, and sexual orientation, which I didn't fully understand then. Before I even knew I liked men, I was called "a faggot," "a cocksucker." Before I even had a theoretical grasp on my identity, other classmates would put me in a box, objectify me, and dominate me. That violence hurt me. And it's this pain that traverses *Quelqu'un*: that of having been depersonalized before being able to become someone.

KL: I don't know if what we call "Saguenay—Lac-Saint-Jean" is more violent or less violent than other spaces. One thing is certain, though; like the rest of America, this "region" is built upon stolen land, on an inaugural violence. In this sense, one mustn't think of "Saguenay—Lac-Saint-Jean" as this natural, unchanged, and never-changing space. Before 1957, the name didn't even exist. Still today, governments and international firms just consider it a vast space to extract resources. This territory carves out a zone at the confluence of two traditional territories: that of the Innus and the Hurons-Wendats. Imperial cartography has erased them.

For historical reasons, this region has a rather open relationship with homophobia, transphobia, but also with anti-Indigenous racism, and more generally, "the fear of the Other." There are several reasons for this, and I cannot name them all. The family was a central force in the colonial enterprise, and gay people and "foreigners," notably, were thought to be breaking family transmission. The fact that LGBTQ+ individuals often leave the region for big cities makes the intergenerational transmission and support difficult at the local level (lots of people commit suicide; in 2020 alone three of my acquaintances died). Overall, it doesn't interest me much to say that "the region is violent," more so than elsewhere (which I doubt it is). It's above all a sort of archeology and willingness to understand the complexities and nuances of a situation that push me to write.

JA & LB: Your texts make room for (naked and sexualized) bodies, for bodily fluids, and their consumption. Is there for you a difference between pleasure and desire? To what extent does pornography influence your representations?

NG: I would say that desire is the starting point of everything, feeling a man's spark, seeing a body that turns me on. Pleasure is what comes after. It's the product of desire, the result of consuming desire. Pornography certainly influences the variations of these desires and these pleasures. Like many other young gays—who live in rural places—pornography was my first source of, albeit distorting, representations of male homosexuality. I use "distorting" because I soon realized that pornography was a vehicle for a whole host of stereotypes (racist ones, among others), violence, and that it wasn't a true "reflection" of gay sexuality, which is so much richer and complex than the hackneyed scenario: foreplay, naked bodies, oral sex, anal sex, ejaculation, sharing of bodily fluids. Sexuality, whichever it may be, is not a narrative schema or a set pattern to follow. It's why I try to distance myself more and more from this imaginary, even if I recognize that it still influences me; my books are clearly very explicit.

KL: In *Querelle . . .* , I wanted to write a type of sexual consumption that is widespread today, produced most notably by hookup applications and pornography. Desire for me, like for Nicholas, is a sort of general starting point. Desire is the name of that energy that leads us towards others. Desire, as I understand it, is never a singular thing. It's always made up of contrary currents, of opposing desires. We always want one thing and the other. What interests me is that an entire part of desire is anchored today in a *neoliberal* logic of consumption and desire. As Deleuze, Guattari, and Hocquenghem have shown, the most capitalist version of desire hinges on a logic of *lack,* which is connected to buying power. That's why in *Querelle de Roberval*, my main character, Querelle, is in love with several men, never with just one, because a single person never fills the fundamental lack that the capitalist logic places on the individual. I wanted to explore this knot between economy and libido.

JA & LB: Is the intertextual dimension of your writing part of an attempt at relationality, interlinking? Considering the references, do you consider yourself part of a lineage of rawness?

NG: Intertextuality is clearly a key element to my writing. I use it in all its forms: direct or indirect citations, allusions, paraphrases, approximations, permutations, etc. It's impossible for me to write without my "mental libraries and catalogs." I am part of the raw lineage because I cite sexually explicit literary works. I think for instance of the epigraph to *Queues*, which is an ode to Jean-Paul Daoust's amazing collection *Black Diva.* It's also because I'm very easily inspired by mainstream culture and viral references. So, rock music, Hollywood cinematographic productions, and TV series all fuel my imagination. This double intertextuality makes my writing rawer, I think. It is a heterogeneous, hybrid, raw, and enriching intertextuality.

KL: Queer intertextuality is linked to the question of "transmission," a word I do not like because it hinges on the heterosexual family and the inheritance of financial assets. Let's say that the relationship to other texts allows me to think about certain realities for a more extended period of time, to learn from those who preceded me and who are sometimes ahead of me, who also inform me of possible futures (it isn't strictly a matter of chronology). Queer cultures are not institutionalized so there is no official form of transmission. As such, the question of the relationship between generations is also complex; no institution means no dialogue or continuity. Queer works are more quickly forgotten for this reason; they usually follow logics that are different from pre-established processes of "transmission," often copied from the hetero, even patriarchal, notion of transmission. Other authors allow me to break the solitude and confinement in the present and to imagine another mode of relationality—with other people, other generations, and other eras—that is not grounded in the concept of "inheritance."

Index

About the Contributors

John Ashburn is a doctoral student in francophone studies at the University of Louisiana at Lafayette where he also received an MA in French. He is currently working on his dissertation which explores contemporary queer literature and screen productions in Quebec.

Loïc Bourdeau is an associate professor of French and francophone studies at the University of Louisiana at Lafayette. His research lies in 20th- and 21st-century global French studies, with a focus on literature and screen studies, gender and queer studies, care studies, and politics. Among others, he has edited *Horrible Mothers. Representation across Francophone North America* (UNP 2019) and *ReFocus: The Films of François Ozon* (EUP 2021). He recently completed *Diversity and Decolonization in French Studies: New Approaches to Teaching* (Palgrave 2022). His current book project, *(Un) Cared For: Womanhood and Healthcare in Contemporary French Literature* (LUP), analyzes patient-carer dynamics in post-2000 women's writing. He launched and serves as series editor of *New Directions in Francophone Studies: Diversity, Decolonization, Queerness* (EUP).

V. Hunter Capps is a postdoctoral fellow and visiting assistant professor at the University at Buffalo. Primarily interested in cultivating queer theories of writing, his research focuses on HIV/AIDS literature in America and France. He is interested in exploring how the AIDS crisis and its cultural productions informed contemporary notions of queerness as it pertains to matters of politics, community, and sex. He is the author of "A Small Movement with a Big Agenda: Robin Campillo's BPM." His forthcoming, co-authored article "SARS-CoV-2 and Discursive Inoculation: Lessons from HIV/AIDS" examines how during the COVID-19 pandemic people have resorted to old tactics of speaking about disease that they believe will protect them from contagion such as the military metaphor and moralizing behavior.

David Caron is professor of French and women's and gender studies at the University of Michigan. He is a scholar of 20th- and 21st-century French literature and culture, with specific interests in queer and HIV studies, as well as Holocaust studies. Some of his recent research has focused on the questions of community and republican universalism, dealing with issues such as the engagement of urban spaces by minoritized groups, the cultural and political uses of "the Republic," representations of collective disasters (AIDS, the Holocaust), masculinity, the concepts of neighborhood and family, etc. He has published a number of single-author monographs, including *The Nearness of Others: Searching for Tact and Contact in the Age of HIV*, and a number of articles and book chapters.

João Florêncio is senior lecturer in history of modern and contemporary art and visual culture at the University of Exeter. A queer cultural theorist of the body, his interdisciplinary research focuses on visual cultures of sexuality, health and illness in relation to wider Western biopolitical, philosophical and technoscientific histories. João's work has been published in journals like *Performance Research*, *Performance Philosophy*, *Sexualities*, *Somatec hnics*, *Porn Studies*, and *Radical History Review*. Between 2019 and 2021, he was the recipient of an Arts and Humanities Research Council (AHRC) Leadership Fellows grant to explore contemporary gay "pig" masculinities in pornographic media and sex cultures. He is the author of *Bareback Porn, Porous Masculinities, Queer Futures: The Ethics of Becoming-Pig* (Routledge, 2020).

CJ Gomolka is associate professor of global French studies at DePauw University. His main area of research and publication is sexuality and gender in 21st-century French and francophone cultural studies. His current book project entitled *To(o) Queer the Nation: Nomenclature, Universalism, and Identity in Contemporary France* examines the links between denomination, universalist ideologies, and identity formation through chapters on the genesis and circulation of *transpédégouine*, the anti-feminicide campaign known as the *colleur-euses* movement, naming censorship on French social media platforms, and the "beyond naming" ideologies of transfeminist activists Paul Preciado and Sam Bourcier. His second book project *Biotechsex: (Sexual) Citizenship, Pharmacoporn Power, and Contemporary France* explores the saturation of the French marketplace with biomedical and pornographic protocols as a dynamic site for the production of novel configurations of queer and non-queer bodies, subjectivities, and citizenship models.

Daniel N. Maroun teaches at the University of Illinois where his primary research interests are gender and sexuality in cultural productions of French expression. One of his larger axes of research is representations of HIV/AIDS in literature and cinema. He co-edited a special issue of *Contemporary French Civilization* (vol. 46, no. 2) that explored the concept of memorialization in both cinematic and literary representations of HIV/AIDS as well as served as translator for Guillaume Dustan's first three novels.

Lucille Toth is an assistant professor of French at the Ohio State University-Newark. Trained in contemporary dance, her research interests lie at the intersection of dance, medical humanities and gender studies. Her first book *Danse et pandémie. Du sida au COVID-19* uses dance to challenge contemporary cultural, political and artistic metaphors of contamination in France and beyond. In addition to being a scholar, Lucille Toth is also a choreographer and the founder of *On Boarder(hers)*, a dance-therapy project welcoming immigrants and documenting their testimonies via movement.

Brian Troth is an HIV/AIDS and French gay culture specialist who earned his PhD from The Ohio State University in 2019. His work confronts filmic and literary interpretations of the HIV epidemic to show the ways in which sexual health and risk have evolved both medically and in how they are perceived by gay men. Dr. Troth's recent work has examined the various ways in which gay men interact via social media and social networking apps, the creation of digital personae, the effects of preventative medicine on sexual practices/perceptions, and gay identity in France. He is currently the gender, sex, and relationships editor for *Synapsis*, a health humanities journal.

www.ingramcontent.com/pod-product-compliance
Ingram Content Group UK Ltd.
Pitfield, Milton Keynes, MK11 3LW, UK
UKHW041838031026
15587UKWH00002B/868

9 781793 650085